Carnivore Mastery: Unleash Your Full Potential

Manha .B Williams

Funny helpful tips:

Your essence is a beacon; shine brightly, guiding others through the darkness.

Engage with autobiographies; they offer firsthand insights into notable individuals' lives and experiences.

Carnivore Mastery: Unleash Your Full Potential : Unlock Your True Power: Master the Art of Carnivorous Eating for Optimal Performance

Life advices:

Stay curious and ask questions; seeking answers drives a deeper understanding of texts.

In the vastness of the universe, find wonder in your existence and purpose in your pursuits.

Introduction

In this guide to the Carnivore Diet, readers are introduced to a unique dietary approach that challenges conventional nutritional wisdom. It begins by laying the groundwork for understanding dieting and nutrients, setting the stage for the exploration of the Carnivore Diet.

The guide defines the Carnivore Diet, highlighting its central principle of excluding plant-based foods entirely. It delves into the scientific basis of this diet, explaining the rationale behind its design and how it differs from mainstream dietary recommendations.

Readers are then presented with an array of health benefits associated with the Carnivore Diet, providing insights into how it may positively impact one's well-being. The guide takes a balanced approach by discussing the potential pros and cons of this diet, dispelling myths and addressing common misconceptions.

To offer a broader perspective, the guide compares the Carnivore Diet to the Ketogenic and Paleo diets, highlighting the key distinctions among these dietary approaches. It also addresses the shortcomings of conventional diets, shedding light on why they may not always be effective.

For practical implementation, readers discover a list of allowed foods on the Carnivore Diet along with their nutritional values, equipping them with the knowledge needed for success. The guide offers valuable tips on how to thrive on this diet, emphasizing the importance of planning and preparation.

Cost-conscious individuals will appreciate the section on saving money while following the Carnivore Diet. Additionally, those interested in building muscle on this diet will find useful information, including tips for achieving their fitness goals.

The guide concludes with a comprehensive FAQ section, addressing common queries and concerns that readers may have. It further enhances the reader's experience by providing a collection of enticing recipes for red meat, white meat, seafood, and organ meats, making it easier to incorporate the Carnivore Diet into their daily lives.

In essence, this guide serves as a comprehensive resource for beginners looking to explore the Carnivore Diet. It offers valuable insights, practical tips, and a diverse range of recipes, enabling individuals to embark on their carnivorous dietary journey with confidence and knowledge.

Contents

INTRODUCTION TO THE CARNIVORE DIET

DIETING AND NUTRIENTS

The term "diet" generally refers to the set of foods a person eats. However, diet can also mean food and meals designed to achieve certain therapeutic effects. The foods we eat provide our body with the nutrients it needs to grow and function properly.

These nutrients are:

Carbohydrates. They are macro (big) nutrients and they provide the body with energy (fuel) needed for our daily activities and also for the different processes that go on in the body. Sources of carbohydrates include rice, oatmeal, yam, potatoes, and cassava.

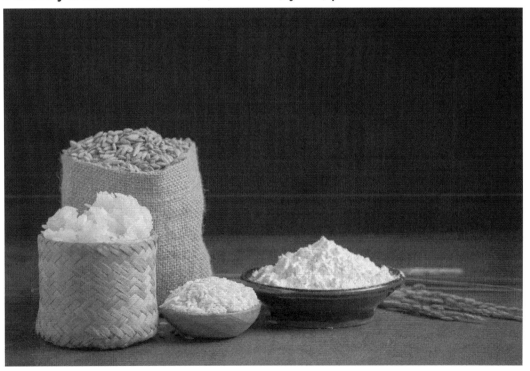

Proteins. They are also macro molecules like carbohydrates. They help to repair worn out tissues in the body. They also help in growth. Proteins can be obtained from foods of animal origin (meat, fish and eggs), as well as some vegetable sources of food such as soybeans, peanuts, almonds, peanuts, lentils.

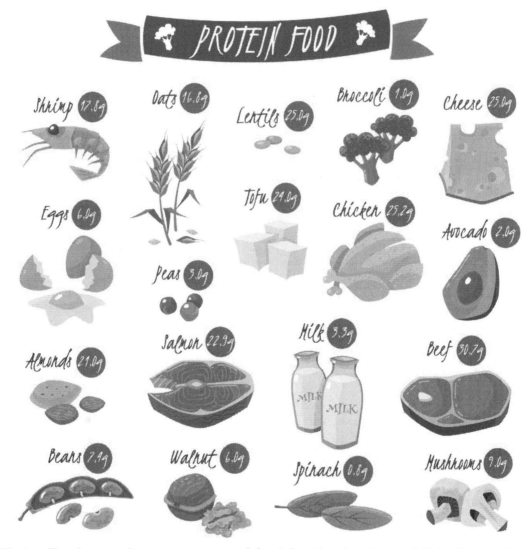

Fats. Fat is used as a source of fuel for the body and it is the major way the body stores energy. Fat also serve as a carrier medium for some vitamins (vitamin A, vitamin D, vitamin E, vitamin K). Fat can be obtained from foods like nuts, cheese, pork, and avocado, fatty fish and so on.

Vitamins. Vitamins are nutrients that the body needs in small amounts to grow and function effectively. There are two classes of vitamins: fat-soluble and water-soluble. Fat-soluble vitamins are vitamins A, D, E, and K. They are present in foods containing fats. The body absorbs these vitamins as it does dietary fats. They do not dissolve in water. Water-soluble vitamins are carried to the body's tissues but are not stored in the body. They are found in many plant and animal foods and in dietary supplements and must be taken in daily. The water-soluble vitamins include ascorbic acid (vitamin C), thiamin, riboflavin, niacin, vitamin B6 (pyridoxine, pyridoxal, and pyridoxamine), folacin, vitamin B12, biotin, and pantothenic acid.

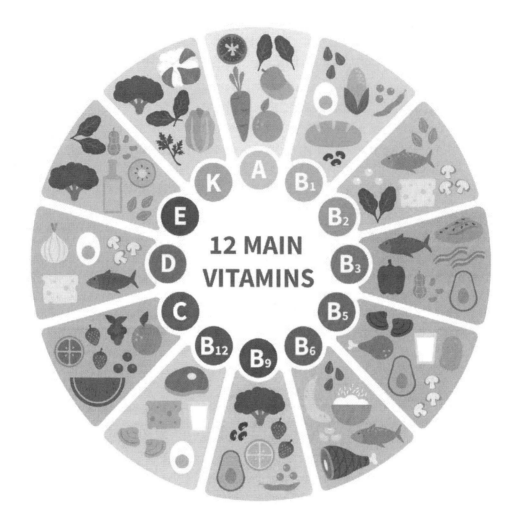

Minerals. Minerals are essential nutrients needed by the body in small quantity. They have diverse functions in the body ranging from ensuring strong bones to wound healing and ensuring blood clotting. Examples of minerals are calcium, phosphorus, magnesium, iron, iodine etc. They can be found in fruits and vegetables, palm oil, organ meat etc.

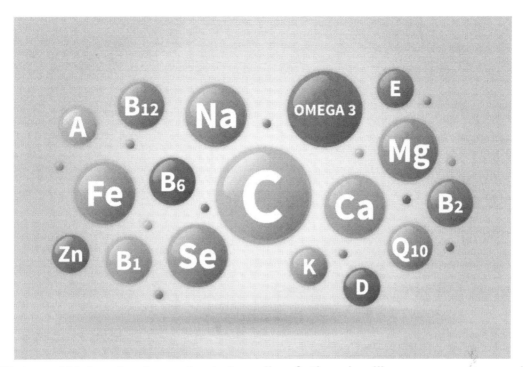

Water. Water is important in all of the bodily processes and functions. It is present in almost every food item and it helps to maintain the temperature of the body. It also serves a means of transport for nutrients in the body.

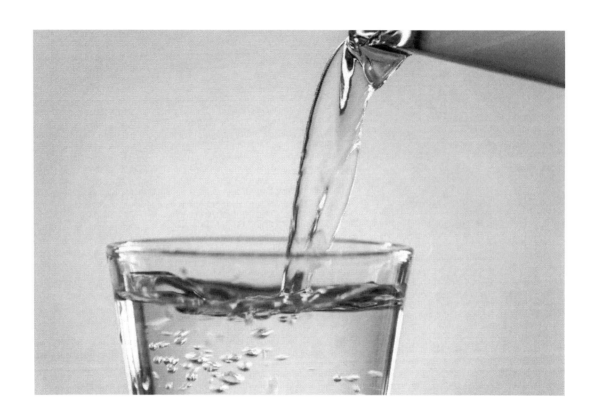

WHAT IS THE CARNIVORE DIET

The carnivore diet is an elimination diet that involves the consumption of only foods of animal origin. Being devoid of any plant food source, the carnivore diet is rich in proteins and fats contained in meat and low (or practically free) in carbohydrates. It is basically a more extreme variant of the ketogenic diet.

People often try the carnivore diet after trying the paleo diet or the ketogenic diet to lose body fat. The carnivore diet is in some ways similar to the ketogenic diet and the paleo diet, but is different in that instead of eating vegetables, meat and oil as in the ketogenic diet, and instead of eating only a variety of plant-based foods such as fruits and vegetables as in the paleo diet, the carnivore diet allows you to eat only meat. In the carnivore diet, carbohydrate intake is practically zero because there is no plant-based food intake at all.

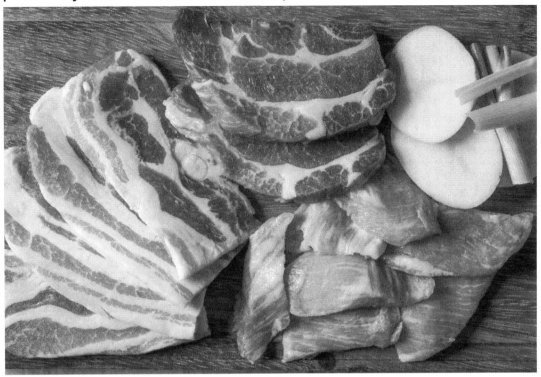

No plant foods means that cereals, roots, fruits, vegetables, nuts, seeds and legumes are not allowed. Also, tea and coffee are limited because they are of plant origin. Seasonings are also limited, but salt and pepper are allowed in small quantities.

A typical carnivore diet includes meat (of all types: red meat, lean meat, beef, pork, bacon, lamb, and so on), organ meat (such as brain, liver, heart, kidney, gizzard, etc.), fish (of all kinds imaginable), poultry (chicken, turkey, duck, guinea fowl and any other bird that can be eaten by man), eggs (of all kinds), bone marrow, bone broth, lard and tallow. In extreme cases, the carnivore diet includes only meat (of various types) and water.

MAIN BENEFITS OF THE CARNIVORE DIET

- Weight loss
- Improved appetite control
- Improved digestion
- Improved mental clarity
- Increased level of testosterone
- Improved mood
- Healing from food allergies
- Reduced inflammation
- Good heart health
- Muscle gain

To learn more about these and many other benefits, consult the chapter Health Benefits Of The Carnivore Diet.

HOw DOES THE CARNIVORE DIET WORK

The carnivore diet works through two major mechanisms:

- It restricts the nutrients that are not needed and that cause autoimmune diseases.
- It replaces restricted nutrients with nutrients needed for weight loss, immunomodulation and other functions.

With regards to weight loss, a major way the carnivore diet works is by helping people to eat less food. This is possible because proteins are satiating (causing someone to feel full with little amount eaten). Even though meat tastes delicious, there is a very low probability of eating too much, unlike when eating snacks or desserts like doughnuts or ice cream. So, this lesser food intake caused by the feeling of satiety leads to a reduction in calories intake.

Furthermore, the carnivore diet favors weight loss by making the body go into ketosis, a metabolic state where the body is using fat to generate energy instead if using carbohydrates for the same purpose. While using fat as a source of energy, one can't get spikes in insulin so the body cannot store excess fat as body fat.

BASIC CARNIVORE DIET FOOD LIST

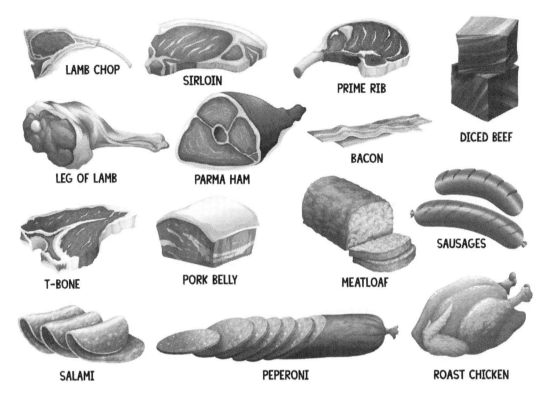

LAMB CHOP   SIRLOIN   PRIME RIB   DICED BEEF

LEG OF LAMB   PARMA HAM   BACON

T-BONE   PORK BELLY   MEATLOAF   SAUSAGES

SALAMI   PEPERONI   ROAST CHICKEN

Meat: Bacon, pork, ham, lamb, beef, steak. High-fat meats are recommended because, being the carnivore a zero-carbohydrate diet, fat must be supplied to the body as a source of energy.

Fish: Catfish, mackerel fish, sardine, salmon, trout and basically any high-fat fish.

Eggs: Any bird's eggs can be eaten. Eggs help provide essential vitamins and also the minerals needed by the body for its proper functioning.

Fats and oils: Animal-based fats such as tallow and lard should be used in cooking when following the carnivore diet. Again, it is important not to use vegetable oils.

Dairy products: Dairy products, such as milk and cheese, should be consumed in minimal quantities or, better yet, excluded entirely.

Bone Marrow: Bone marrow is an excellent source of protein that can be taken on the carnivore diet.

Seasonings: Be careful to choose seasonings that do not contain sugar or carbohydrates. Examples of seasonings that can be chosen include pepper, salt and spices, among others.

Snacks. Example of snacks allowed while on the carnivore diet are:

- Jerky stick
- Pork rinds
- Bacon snacks
- Meat snacks
- Tuna
- Salami snacks
- Salmon snacks
- Chicken salad
- Pork salad
- Crab
- Snails
- Sushi
- Meat stick

THE ORIGINS OF THE CARNIVORE DIET

There is historical evidence that some ancient peoples had a primarily carnivorous diet, although over time these civilizations also consumed plant-based foods when available. These populations and groups are:

- **Masai, Rendille and Samburu of East Africa**: their diet was mainly composed of meat of all kinds and milk. The young male population ate almost exclusively all of these foods of animal origin, but also occasionally consumed herbs and bark when available. The women and men of the older generations consumed fruit, honey and even tubers.

- **The nomads of Mongolia**: they ate mainly meat and dairy products, but also got nutrients from the consumption of wild onions and garlic, tubers and roots, seeds and berries.
- **The Canadian Inuit**: These people mainly subsisted on whale meat, fish, seals and walruses, but also went to great lengths to search for and harvest sea vegetables, lichens and berries for their consumption. They have even gone so far as to employ the fermentation technique in the processing of some of these plant-based foods as a way to store them for future use.
- **Gaucho Brazilians**: These people consumed mostly beef, but they supplemented their diet with yerba mate, an herbal infusion rich in vitamins, minerals, and phytonutrients.
- **The Russian Arctic Chukotka**: They fed majorly on fish, caribou, and marine animals, but they always ate them with local roots, leafy greens, berries, or seaweed.
- **The Sioux of South Dakota**: They fed on large amounts of buffalo meat majorly, but they also ate seeds, nuts and the wild fruits that they found as they followed the buffalo herds.

It is important to note that each of these above-mentioned populations ate some plant foods at certain times, thus adopting a combination of plant and animal food sources in their diets. This fact does not mean that the carnivore diet is inadequate and that plants are necessary to stay healthy, but it is interesting in that it shows those populations' wisdom in balancing things.

WHY "NO PLANTS" IS BETTER

PLANTS CONTAIN ANTI-NUTRIENTS

Plants are excluded from the carnivore diet because they contain anti-nutrients. Anti-nutrients are compounds that reduce the digestion and absorption of nutrients by our body. Examples of anti-nutrients are:

Tannins: they are a class of polyphenols which have anti-oxidative effects and impair the digestion and absorption of many minerals.

Protease inhibitors: this category of anti-nutrients inhibits digestive enzymes, which negatively affects the digestion of proteins. They are found in a wide range of plants from grains to legumes to even seeds. An example of protease inhibitors is Bowman which inhibits pepsin, trypsin and other proteases which are present in the gut. This prevents the digestion and also the absorption of proteins and amino acids.

Phytic acid: this is also known as phylate and it hinders absorption of certain minerals such as zinc, iron, calcium and magnesium. They are present in grains, seeds and legumes.

Lectins: they are harmful in high levels and they hinder absorption of nutrients. They can be found in all plant sources of food.

Lipase inhibitors: they are compounds found in plant that inhibit the hydrolysis of certain lipids by interfering with the enzymes that catalyze the hydrolysis of those lipids (lipase). Examples of lipid inhibitors are simvastatin, pitavastatin, lovastatin, rosuvastatin, atorvastatin, fluvastatin and pravastatin.

Calcium oxalate: calcium oxalate is the primary form in which calcium is present in many vegetables. This form of calcium is not absorbed well by the body and it is present in spinach, peanut, beetroot.

Amylase inhibitors: amylase inhibitors prevent the release and absorption of simple sugars in the body by preventing enzymatic actions that break the glycosidic bonds present in complex carbohydrates like starch. When this happens, simple sugars are not released for use into the body.

PLANTS ARE A CAUSE OF FOOD ALLERGIES

Plants are the most occurring causes of food allergy and some cross reactive syndromes. In plants, a substantial part of allergens have defense-related function and their expression is highly influenced by environmental stress and diseases. Pathogenesis-related proteins (PR) account for about 25% of plant food allergens and some are responsible for extensive cross-reactions between plant-derived foods, pollen and latex allergens.

PLANT FOODS INTAKE FAVORS WEIGHT GAIN

Plants are a major source of carbohydrates, which can lead to weight gain if consumed in excess. This is because the body stores excess glucose as body fat, which adds to fat tissue and ultimately leads to weight gain. This does not happen in the carnivore diet because foods of plant origin are totally excluded. The body synthesizes the glucose it needs from meat, which is high in protein and essentially free of carbohydrates, through a process called gluconeogenesis (more on that later).

THE SCIENTIFIC BASIS OF THE CARNIVORE DIET

The scientific basis of the efficacy of the carnivore diet has its roots in the concepts of ketosis and gluconeogenesis. Glucose is stored in our liver and released when needed for energy. However, if carbohydrate intake has been low for a while (say a day or two), these glucose stores are depleted, the body enters ketosis and initiates gluconeogenesis to produce the energy it needs. Gluconeogenesis occurs when the liver produces glucose from the amino acids of the ingested protein, while ketosis is the process by which the body synthesizes glucose from fats instead of carbohydrates.

KETOSIS

Ketosis is a metabolic state in which high levels of ketone bodies are present in the blood or urine. It is a normal response of the body when the glucose level is low or unavailable. This condition occurs when an individual is on special diets such as low-carb diets or when fasting. Ketosis is a mechanism for providing an additional source of energy for the brain in the form of ketones.

The level of carbohydrate restriction required to induce people into a state of ketosis is not constant, it is variable and depends on many factors such as an individual's level of physical activity, level of insulin sensitivity, genetics and age, but ketosis usually occurs when you are consuming less than 50 grams of carbohydrates per day for about three days. This is exactly what happens while on the carnivore diet. Ketosis can also be induced by the consumption of ketogenic fats (such as medium-chain triglycerides) or by the consumption of exogenous ketones in foods or supplements.

Ketosis can be measured by urinalysis, serum analysis, and blood work. Urine testing is the most common method for ketone testing. The urine test strips use a nitroprusside reaction principle with acetoacetate to provide a semi-quantitative measurement based on the color change of the strip. Although beta-hydroxybutyrate is the predominant circulating ketone, urine test strips only measure acetoacetate. Urinary ketones are often poorly correlated with serum levels due to variability in the excretion of ketones by the kidneys, the influence of hydration status and renal function. The breath test can be conducted using some portable devices that have already been set up to measure ketosis by measuring acetone as an estimate.

Ketosis has some major medical implications.

- **Treatment of epilepsy.** Ketosis is used in the treatment of epilepsy. It was first used to treat epilepsy in the 1920s and is now widely accepted and implemented in both the treatment of pediatric patients and the treatment of adult patients.
- **Management of obesity.** Ketosis, as a result of low-carb diets, has been shown to be effective in managing obesity and promoting weight loss. Ketosis improves some markers of metabolic syndrome by reducing serum triglycerides, increasing high-density lipoprotein (HDL), and increasing the size and volume of low-density lipoprotein (LDL) particles. These changes are consistent with an improved lipid profile despite potential increases in total cholesterol level.
- **Treatment of type 2 diabetes.** Ketosis induced by low carbohydrate diets has been supported as a treatment that has been shown to be effective in the management of type 2 diabetes, because it helps to reduce dietary glucose load and this increases the sensitivity of insulin and hemoglobin and it also reduces the need for exogenous insulin. However, people with pancreatitis should not be on any diet that induces ketogenesis due to the high dietary fat content. For the same reason, people with fat metabolism disorders should not be on any diet that can induce ketogenesis.

GLUCONEOGENESIS

Gluconeogenesis is the production of glucose from sources that are not carbohydrate in nature. It is the production of new glucose (i.e. synthesis of glucose from sources other than glycogen). This synthesis is from substrates produced by the breakdown of protein (glycogenic amino acids), break down of lipids (triglycerides) and pyruvate and lactate. This metabolic process is one of the mechanisms used by the body to maintain an adequate level of glucose in the blood and to prevent hyperglycemia.

Gluconeogenesis is very important for the body. It is important to make glucose available even in the absence of carbohydrates in order to prevent hypoglycemia. Hypoglycemia is a condition where the human body has a low glucose level. The human body requires a very constant supply of glucose especially for the nervous system and also for the erythrocytes (the most common type of blood cells and the vertebrate's principal means of delivering oxygen (O_2) to the body tissues—via blood flow through the circulatory system).

Hypoglycemia causes brain dysfunction, which in most cases leads to coma and even death. Another important function of glucose is to maintain adequate concentrations of citric acid cycle intermediates even when fatty acids are the main source of acetyl-CoA in tissues. Furthermore, gluconeogenesis eliminates lactate produced by muscles and erythrocytes and glycerol produced by adipose tissue. In ruminants, propionate is a product of rumen carbohydrate metabolism and is an important substrate for gluconeogenesis.

Excessive gluconeogenesis occurs in critically ill patients in response to injury and infection, contributing to hyperglycemia which is associated with an unfavorable outcome. Hyperglycemia leads to changes in the osmolality of body fluids, impaired blood flow, intracellular acidosis and increased production of superoxide radicals, resulting in impaired endothelial and immune system function and impaired blood clotting. Excessive gluconeogenesis is also a contributing factor to hyperglycemia in type 2 diabetes due to impaired regulation in response to insulin.

HEALTH BENEFITS OF THE CARNIVORE DIET

WEIGHT LOSS

The carnivore diet is effective for losing weight primarily because it puts the body into ketosis, a metabolic state in which fats are used to generate energy instead of carbohydrates. While using fat as an energy source there can be no insulin spikes, so the body cannot store excess fat in the form of body fat.

Another major reason the carnivore diet is beneficial for weight loss is that it helps people eat less food. This is because the proteins are very filling. Even though the meat tastes delicious there is a very low chance of overeating, unlike with snacks or desserts such as donuts or ice cream. Thus, the reduced food intake caused by the feeling of satiety leads to a reduction in calories.

Additionally, studies on the carnivore diet have shown that it has the ability to suppress appetite because it contains a combination of very high protein and little or no sugar. Appetite suppression acts by direct influence on major hunger-causing hormones such as leptin and ghrelin. Additionally, lack of dietary diversity (food monotony, which consists of eating one type of food over and over) has been shown to reduce calorie intake. When the same food is presented to us often, the level of interest the food provokes decreases, resulting in less food consumption and less likelihood of overeating. That is why when following the carnivore diet there is no need to count calorie intake or monitor food consumption. Since calorie counting is not absolutely necessary, you can eat your fill without fear of getting too many calories.

IMPROVED DIGESTION

By excluding the intake of plants, the carnivore diet helps reduce bloating and also helps reduce and prevent some digestive disorders. This is because the lectins and some anti-nutrients that are present in some plants most often irritate the gastrointestinal tract and lead to digestive disorders.

IMPROVED MENTAL CLARITY

People on the carnivore diet claim it helps in reducing brain fog and that it helps in improving their cognitive function. They also claim to experience much more clarity and a greater sense of calmness than when they were on high carb diet. This is because a diet of meat, high in protein and low in carbohydrates, helps to improve the reaction time.

BETTER ENERGY AND SLEEP

People on the carnivore diet are reported to have better energy and better sleeping patterns. The intake of meat increases the branched chain amino acids and the phenylalanine in the blood. The branched chain amino acid helps in the reduction of fatigue.

HEALING FROM FOOD ALLERGIES

Plants are the main causes of food allergy because they contain leptin and some other anti-nutrients that can be allergens. Since the carnivore diet is highly restrictive of non-animal foods, it helps prevent food allergies because potentially allergic foods are simply not allowed. People allergic to many foods will likely find trying the carnivore diet especially helpful.

REDUCED AUTOIMMUNE CONDITIONS

The carnivore diet has been shown to reduce autoimmune conditions like type 1 diabetes, inflammatory bowel diseases, and chronic inflammatory demyelinating polyneuropathy. This is because lections and certain anti nutrients which are present in some vegetables most times aggravate autoimmune conditions and contribute to pains. Furthermore, the meat diet (another name for the carnivore diet) works to affect autoimmunity by restricting calories and fasting. Auto immunity is a condition in which immune responses are misdirected and the immune system starts to attack its own cells and tissues instead of attacking foreign cells that evade the body. Diseases caused by auto immunity are called auto immune disease. Examples of auto immune diseases are type 1 diabetes, rheumatoid arthritis, celiac disease, pernicious anemia, Graves' disease and vitiligo.

In addition, the carnivore diet works to alter the gut microbiota as a result of the intermittent fasting associated with the diet. Intermittent fasting has effects that are potentially immunomodulatory in nature. Immunomodulation is the modulation of the immune system to prevent and control autoimmunity. The gut microbiota is linked to immunity according to some studies. In one of those studies, patients with multiple sclerosis (a type of autoimmune disease) were treated with minocycline (an antibiotic which clears bad bacteria from the gut so as to improve the symptoms of multiple sclerosis) and the positive effects were seen and they lasted for a while. The carnivore diet has these same effects because it helps to clear the bacteria from the gut. Although this might have undesirable effects because it clears both good and bad bacteria from the gut.

REDUCED INFLAMMATION

The carnivore diet helps in reduction of inflammation in some people because it is high in fat. The liver produces C-reactive proteins (CRP) in response to inflammation, so measuring CRP levels can indicate how much inflammation is in your system. A level of 10mg/L or less is normal, and 1mg/L or less is good. Restring the intake of foods from animal sources actually helps to reduce the rate if inflammation because many people are sensitive to some foods from plant sources. The lower inflammation rate helps to reduce, prevent and manage pains that arise from inflammation.

REDUCED AUTISM SYMPTOMS

The carnivore diet is highly inclusive of substances that help in reducing the symptoms of autism and highly exclusive of substances that worsen autism symptoms. Meat naturally has a high level of cysteine present in it. Cysteine is an amino acid that has been shown overtime to reduce the symptoms of autism. N-acetylcysteine (NAC) is a compound that functions by releasing cysteine helped in the reduction of irritability which is normally associated with autism conditions in multiple trials.

As a result of the fact that every food allowed in the carnivore diet contains a very high level of cysteine, this diet is definitely much higher in cysteine than the average normal diet. In addition, meat has very high levels of carnitine. A research work found out that children who have autism also have low levels of carnitine and another research study found out that that carnitine supplements helps to reduce symptoms compared to the placebo group.

Increased intake of omega-3 fatty acids has also improved symptoms of autism, though some people responded better than others to supplementation. Oily fish (like salmon and sardines) are rich in omega-3 fatty acids. Zinc, which is abundant in meat, can increase regulatory T cells (Tregs) and benefit people with autoimmunity. Zinc supplements have even improved symptoms in some people who have autism.

GLAUCOMA PREVENTION

Vitamin B3 (nicotinamide) is found naturally in foods from animal sources and it helps to prevent and also to treat glaucoma, a disease condition of the eye in which the nerve that connects the eye to the brain gets damaged. This is most times due to a high pressure of the eye and it can lead to blindness if not properly treated.

INCREASED LEVEL OF TESTOSTERONE

Men who follow this high fat diet have the probability of having a higher testosterone level. A study in the American Journal of Clinical Nutrition found that men who followed a high-fat, low-fiber diet for 10 weeks had 13% higher total testosterone than subjects who ate low fat and high fiber.

RICH IN MICRONUTRIENTS

The carnivore diet grants intake of important micronutrients. Liver is a rich source of vitamin A, Vitamin D, foliate and choline. The carnivore diet gives room for adequate intake of liver in meals, therefore one can be sure to get and have an adequate supply of these nutrients on this diet. In the same vein, oysters and salmon are rich in iron, iodine, vitamin D, copper, selenium, manganese and also in omega 3 fatty acids, and this diet give room for adequate consumption of these nutrients. Moreover, the nutrients in meat are bioavailable. They require very little or no conversion for the body to start using them because they are already in animal form compared to nutrients from plant food sources, which need to be converted into forms that can be used by the body.

NO PROCESSED FOODS

By restricting food intake to basically only meat and water, the carnivore diet prevents the intake of unhealthy and potentially harmful foods (such as processed foods, which are known to be harmful to the human body).

NO PESTICIDES

Not only the carnivore diet prevents the intake of phytonutrients in plants, but also prevents the consumption of plants contaminated or poisoned by pesticides used to treat them on the farm.

PROS, CONS, MYTHS AND MISCONCEPTIONS

THE PROS OF THE CARNIVORE DIET

- There is no confusion as to what to eat and what not to eat: carnivore diet = meat + water.
- There is no need to track calorie intake and monitor food consumption.
- While on the carnivore diet you can eat to your fill, as much as you want and as many times as you want, without the risk of gaining weight.
- A high-protein diet like the carnivore diet is very filling, so it's nearly impossible to overeat.
- A diet rich in protein and low in carbohydrates such as the carnivore diet helps reduce appetite by intervening at the hormonal level.
- The lack of dietary diversity results in less food intake, thus reducing the level of calorie intake.
- Reduction of brain fog and improved cognitive function are associated with the carnivore diet due to the low carbohydrate content.
- People on the carnivore diet are reported to have better energy and better sleeping patterns.
- The carnivore diet helps to reduce bloating and also helps to reduce and prevent certain symptoms of digestive disorders.
- The carnivore diet can act as an immunomodulating agent thanks to the intermittent fasting that occurs due to satiety.
- The carnivore diet helps prevent and treat food allergies due to its restrictive nature.
- The level of inflammation is significantly reduced with the carnivore diet. This in turn helps reduce pain, especially in

the joints.

- Symptoms of autism are reduced in people following the carnivore diet.
- The carnivore diet helps to prevent and also to treat glaucoma.
- The carnivore diet grants intake of important micronutrients.
- This carnivore diet prevents the intake of phytonutrients in plants and also prevents the consumption of plants contaminated or poisoned by pesticides used to treat them on the farm.
- The carnivore diet prevents the intake of unhealthy and potentially harmful foods, such as processed foods.

POSSIBLE CONS

Here are the most common objections to the carnivore diet you should be aware of before starting the diet. I also dedicated the next section to the most common Myths & Misconceptions about the carnivore diet, where you may find answer to several of the following objections. You should always consult your doctor or medical professional of choice before beginning any food regimen. My suggestion is to make your own opinion on the carnivore diet by getting as much information as possible, not limited to this book, and trying it for yourself for at least 4 weeks under the eye of a health professional you trust.

- There is not much scientific research to support the carnivore diet.
- There is little or no research studies about the safety of the carnivore diet.
- Eating only meat and water might be very difficult to abide by.

- The diet might be expensive for people to follow strictly. I provide 6 tips to save money on the carnivore diet in a later chapter.
- Because of the strict meal plan (meat and water), having food in other places apart from home can pose a bit of a challenge.
- This diet may lead to a lower level of the serotonin in the brain.
- The carnivore diet does not make for dietary diversity.
- In this diet, the risk of having diseases related to deficiency of nutrients is high.
- In this diet, there is too much intake of protein and the excess protein that is not used by the body is excreted through the liver. Because there is excess protein on this diet, too much stress can be put on the liver and this can lead to disease conditions of the liver.
- The diet may increase the stress of oxidation in the body.
- The diet does not contain certain compounds that are found in plants and are very healthy. Examples of these plant compounds are fiber and also polyphenols.
- It may cause a deregulation of the gut microbiota if taken for long.
- The carnivore diet may not be healthy in the long term because it lacks some minerals, vitamins and trace elements necessary for the cells and tissues of the human body to function as they should.
- There is a risk of developing colon cancer when on the carnivore diet. This is because anti-oxidants which are present in fruits and vegetables help to prevent and fight carcinogenic substances in the body and since they're not consumed in the carnivore diet, there is a potentially high risk of developing colon cancer.

MYTHS & MISCONCEPTIONS

The common myths and misconceptions about the carnivore diet are listed below in no particular order.

MYTH #1: Plant based food sources (that can be substituted by meat) are healthier than meat.

FACT: Most of those nutrients found in plant-based foods that can be substituted for meat are actually similar to those found in meat. Also, a downside to plant-based sources compared to their meat-based alternatives is that, like many other foods that are ultra-processed, they can cause a higher calorie intake and, as a result, cause weight gain.

MYTH #2: Red meat causes harm to the health of an individual.

FACT: Recent studies (long term observational research) of cancers, diseases of the heart and even death in relation to factors that puts the body at risk like glucose in the blood, cholesterol level of the blood and also inflammation showed that consumption in modest amount of red meat that is not processed is actually neutral for health. Also, meat contains reasonable amounts of certain vitamins and minerals that are essential to the body e.g. Vitamin B complex, Iron, Magnesium and Zinc.

MYTH #3: Beef (cattle) that was grass fed is better for the health.

FACT: Even though 'grass fed' beef sounds like it is a better option, there are no studies yet on the effects of the intake of grass fed beef over conventional fed beef. Conventional fed beef (cattle) eats forage, grain and hay. Forage includes mainly grass. Grass fed cattle would mean that the diet of the cattle is mainly grass.

MYTH #4: If I'm on the carnivore diet, I would have vitamin deficiencies.

FACT: Certain vitamins are present in foods from animal sources. Vitamin C is present in liver, eggs and also in certain fishes. Five of the vitamin B complex (Vitamin B6, VitaminB12, Niacin, Thiamin, Riboflavin) are present meat. Also, vitamin A, vitamin E and vitamin K are present in eggs.

MYTH #5: Intake of meat will definitely cause cancer.

FACT: There is only limited evidence from epidemiological studies that show that a relationship exists between the consumption of meat and cancer. Even in these limited evidences, it has been shown that exposure to other factors like genetics, tobacco smoking, alcohol smoking are risk factors in developing cancer from meat diet.

MYTH #6: Meat is expensive.

FACT: Despite a slight increase in the price of meat relative to the price of plant based foods, we currently spend just 6% of our disposable income on food. Within that 6%, around 21% of our budgets go towards meat. That sounds high until you consider the 31% of grocery expense that went on meat back in 1980. In reality, our efficient meat production system allows us to produce meat for less than ever before.

MYTH #7: Animals are aware of slaughter and they are afraid of it.

FACT: A research carried out by an animal welfare expert named Temple Grandin, Ph.D. found that cows behaved the same whether they are attending a veterinary clinic visit or they are attending a processing plant. Also, pigs had no increase in their heart rate after they saw other pigs slaughtered. Other studies suggest that the symptoms of distress are related more to conditions/factors like presence of noise, lights and some unknown sensations such as blowing of air.

MYTH #8: Antibiotics are primarily used for growth promotion.

FACT: Only about 13% of the antibiotics which are used in agriculture are actually used for the purpose of growth promotion in livestock.

MYTH #9: The use of anti-biotic in animal production is really increasing and it is posing health risks to human beings.

FACT: Antibiotics have been used to treat and prevent illness in animals for a long while, but growing concerns can make it seem like antibiotic use in on the rise. In truth, the FDA efforts we've mentioned to ban growth promotion antibiotics are, in them, proof against this myth. What's more, regulations regarding antibiotics in livestock are stringent. Veterinarians must oversee prescriptions, while withdrawal must take place a set time before slaughter to limit residue in meat. The U.S. Department of Agriculture inspects meat and poultry regularly to ensure these standards. They check both that antibiotic use isn't rising, and that it doesn't pose any health risks.

DIFFERENCES BETWEEN CARNIVORE, KETOGENIC AND PALEO DIET

THE KETO DIET

The keto diet is a diet that is very high in fat; it has adequate protein and is very low in carbohydrate. It is used mainly in managing epilepsy especially in children. It is also used to facilitate weight loss because if its low carb content and high fat content. The keto diet works majorly on the principle of ketosis.

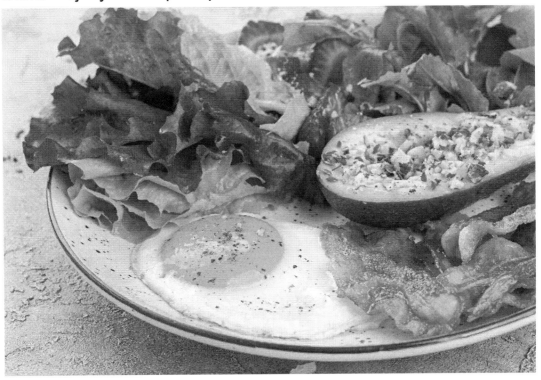

THE PALEO DIET

The paleo diet is based on the principle that the best diet is one that includes only foods that could have been eaten during the Paleolithic, which goes from about 2.5 million to about 10,000 years ago. The paleo diet includes foods that could be the product of hunting and also gathering, such as fruits, nuts, seeds, vegetables, fish and lean meat. The purpose of this diet is basically to get back to what the first men ate.

This is because it is thought that foods obtained from agriculture are not suitable for inclusion in the human diet. Cereals (eg oats, rice, wheat and barley), dairy products (meat, cheese), legumes (peas, beans, peanuts and lentils), sugar, potatoes, salt, and highly processed foods are limited in the paleo diet. The paleo diet can also be used to facilitate weight loss and also to maintain a healthy weight.

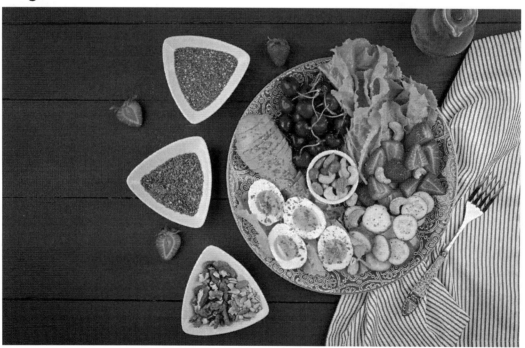

THE THREE DIETS COMPARED

The **similarities** between the carnivore diet, the paleo diet and the keto diet are:

- The paleo diet, carnivore diet and keto diet are all low in carbohydrates.
- All three diets aid in weight loss: Due to their low carb nature, the carnivore diet, paleo diet, and keto diet do not give the body the opportunity to consume carbohydrates, preventing them from being stored as body fat or adipose tissue.

The **differences** between the three diets are:

- The carnivore diet is high in protein and has adequate fat, while the keto diet is high in fat and has adequate protein and the paleo diet is somewhat in between.
- The carnivore diet has zero carbs, while the keto diet functions on a low carb and the paleo diet also functions on a low refined carb principle.
- The carnivore diet is highly restrictive to animal sources of food only unlike the keto diet and the paleo diet.

THE PROBLEMS OF MOST DIETS

- **Short-term effectiveness.** Most of the fad diets don't actually work in the long run. They only work in the short term. A study has shown that about 95% of fad diets no longer work for the intended purpose for which they were started (especially for weight loss) after about 8 months of starting. The same study also showed that about 65% of people who lost weight using a fad diet regained it when they were no longer so strict with the diet. This is because, after losing weight, many people think they have finally reached the end of the journey and are no longer so worried about their diet. This can lead to excessive calorie intake which ends up being stored as fat in the body, contributing to weight gain.

- **Lack of nutrients.** Most diets cause disease due to a lack of certain nutrients that are not present in the diet. This is because fad diets only promote the intake of one type or class of food and limit other types of food or other food classes. In this case, the body cannot get all the nutrients it needs from a type of food or class of food because no single food contains all the nutrients that are essential for the body to function properly. Nutrient deficiency (especially micronutrient deficiency) is a major problem that occurs with most diets.
- **Dehydration.** Fad diets can lead to dehydration in the body. When there is a drop in weight in the body, the excess weight that is lost is not only made up of fat, but also in large part water, which was stored by the body as a reserve to help prevent dehydration. When this water is lost (as a result of most diets), the body runs out of water to use and dehydration sets in. However, this can be avoided by drinking plenty of water every day.
- **Eating out.** Most diets make it difficult or impossible for dieters to eat out (for example at a party, at a friend's house, or simply in a restaurant or take away). This is because there are so many principles and rules about foods to include in your diet and foods not to eat, that eating out becomes very difficult, if not impossible. This could lead to social problems like friends who think you don't like them enough or trust them enough to eat from them, low self-esteem (when you don't even want people to know you're on a diet).
- **Unwelcome psychological effects.** If the diet does not produce the desired results, which prompted one to start

the diet in the first place, one may experience a feeling of defeat which can lead to other unwelcome psychological effects and this can negatively affect the person. Depression may set in, and a lack of satisfaction with one's body may also begin to occur, which can lead to low self-esteem and other social problems.

- **Negative reactions.** Different people can have different reactions to a diet. These reactions could be negative such as irritation of the gastrointestinal tract and this can lead to other disease conditions.
- **Too many rules.** Since most diets contain too many rules, one or more rules may be overlooked and this may make the diet totally ineffective.
- **Lack of principles.** Most diets do not inspire or teach lasting eating habits and actually do not even teach the principle of nutrition. All they do is provide a series of "DOS" and "DONTS" and not necessarily teach the "WHY" of those rules.
- **Unrealistic goals.** Most diets tend to fail because too many unrealistic goals are set in relation to the conditions that can be improved by the diet. When these unrealistic goals are not met, the person following the diet tends to get discouraged and eventually stop the diet.
- **Adaptation problems.** Switching from a regular diet to a new diet causes irritability, mental fog, headaches, confusion and fatigue in most people. This is a big problem with most diets.
- **Binge eating.** Binge eating is also another problem with diets. Binge eating is the habit of eating large amounts of food in one sitting. Binge eating can lead to obesity, a risk factor for many cardiovascular and hormonal diseases. Binge eating occurs with most diets because they don't make certain nutrients available.

- **Calories are everything.** Most diets only focus on calories and leave out other nutrients and classes of food.
- **Ignoring the signals.** Most diets teach the brain to ignore the body. The body actually tells what it needs at a particular time, but dieting teaches you to ignore the body needs and focus on the rules given.
- **Alteration of metabolism.** Most diets affect the normal metabolic rate of the body. They either slow down the rate of metabolism in the body or they quicken it.

WHAT TO EAT: ALLOWED FOODS AND NUTRITIONAL VALUES

In this chapter I am listing several types of meat and other animal foods that can be eaten in the carnivore diet, and their nutritional contents. Remember that in the carnivore diet, to ensure your body all the nutrients it needs, all you have to do is eat your fill of the permitted foods. You don't need to count the calories and the weight of the portions, the beauty of the carnivore diet is just that. However, if in the early days you are in doubt that you are not eating enough and not getting all the essential nutrients into your body, the following information will help you get a better idea of how you are feeding yourself and how the carnivore diet works in your specific case.

Fish & Seafood

Fish are excellent low-carb and high-fat food sources providing a load of extra nutrients, including vitamins, minerals, and fatty acids it is loaded with healthy fats and calories.

Organ Meat

Kidneys, liver, and other organs are extremely rich in nutrients, especially vitamins, minerals, and animal protein but you should also consider bone marrow as it is very tasty and nutritious.

The % Daily Value (DV) tells you how much a nutrient in a serving of food contribute to a daily diet. Note that 2000 calories a day is used for general nutrition advice. Your daily values may be higher or lower depending on your calories needs.

BEEF

Nutritional Value (in 100g)
- Calories: 121

- Total fat: 3 g
- Saturated fat: 1.5 g
- Cholesterol: 60mg
- Protein: 22 g
- Carbohydrate: 0 g
- Sodium: 66 mg
- Vitamin D: 3 mcg
- Iron: 2.44 mg
- Potassium: 357 mg
- Calcium: 8 mg

STEAK

Nutritional Value (in 100g)

- Calories: 221 kilo calories
- Fat: 11.1 g
- Protein: 26g

VEAL

Nutritional Value (in 100g) and % Daily Value*

- Calories 172
- Total Fat 8 g 12%
- Saturated fat 3 g 15%
- Polyunsaturated fat 0.6 g
- Monounsaturated fat 2.8 g
- Cholesterol 103 mg 34%
- Sodium 83 mg 3%
- Potassium 337 mg 9%
- Total Carbohydrate 0 g 0%
- Dietary fiber 0 g 0%
- Sugar g
- Protein 24 g 48%
- Vitamin A 0%

- Vitamin C 0%
- Calcium 1%
- Iron 5%
- Vitamin D 0%
- Vitamin B-6 20%
- Cobalamin 21%
- Magnesium 6%

LIVER

Nutritional Value (in 100g)

- Calorie content: 165
- Protein:26 g
- Total Fat: 4.4 g
- Saturated fat: 1.4 g
- Monounsaturated fat: 0.6 g
- Polyunsaturated fat: 1.1 g
- Cholesterol: 355 g
- Carbohydrate: 3.8 g
- Potassium: 150 mg
- Sodium: 49 mg

PORK

Pork is one of the most popular forms of meat in the whole world and it is classified as red meat because it contains a large amount of myoglobin (a protein responsible for the red color of meat). Pork meat is much cheaper than most other meats.

Pork is a particularly significant source of thiamin (vitamin B1). The content of this important vitamin is much higher than in other meats and that plays and essential role in glucose metabolism and protecting cardiac health.

Pork meat also contains a decent amount of selenium and zinc which are responsible for boosting the immune system, defending against oxidative stress, and optimal hormone production.

Nutritional Value (in 100g) and % Daily Value*

- Calories: 145 calories
- Cholesterol: 80 mg
- Total fat: 14 g (about 21% of the total nutritional content)
- Monounsaturated fat: 6 g
- Polyunsaturated fat: 1.2 g
- Saturated fat: 5 g
- Protein: 27 g (54% of the total nutritional content)
- Total carbohydrate: 0 g
- Sodium: 62 mg
- Potassium: 423 mg
- Vitamin C: 1%
- Vitamin A: 0%
- Iron: 4%
- Magnesium: 7%
- Cobalamin: 11%
- Vitamin B6: 25%
- Calcium: 1%
- Iron: 4%

BACON

Nutritional Value (in 100g)

- Calories: 541 Calories
- Total fat: 42g (about 64% of the nutrients present in beacon)
- Polyunsaturated fat: 4.5 g
- Monounsaturated fat: 19g
- Saturated fat: 14g
- Trans fat: 0g
- Carbohydrate: 1.4 g
- Cholesterol: 110 mg

- Sodium: 1717 mg
- Potassium: 565 mg
- Protein: 37 g (74% of the total nutritional content of bacon)

LAMB

Nutritional Value (in 100g) and % Daily Value*

- Calories 294
- % Daily Value*
- Total Fat 21 g 32%
- Saturated fat 9 g 45%
- Polyunsaturated fat 1.5 g
- Monounsaturated fat 9 g
- Cholesterol 97 mg 32%
- Sodium 72 mg 3%
- Potassium 310 mg 8%
- Total Carbohydrate 0 g 0%
- Dietary fiber 0 g 0%
- Sugar 0 g
- Protein 25 g 50%
- Vitamin A 0%
- Vitamin C 0%
- Calcium 1%
- Iron 10%
- Vitamin D 0%
- Vitamin B-6 5%
- Cobalamin 43%
- Magnesium 5%

CHICKEN

Nutritional Value (in 100g)

- Protein: 27 g

- Total fat: 14 g
- Cholesterol: 88 mg
- Carbohydrate: 9
- Sodium: 82 mg
- Potassium: 223 mg

CHICKEN BROTH

Nutritional Value (in 100g) and % Daily Value*

- Total Fat: 14 g
- Monounsaturated fat: 5 g
- Polyunsaturated fat: 4.5 g
- Saturated fat: 3. 4 g
- Protein: 17 g
- Carbohydrate: 18 g
- Sodium: 23 875 mg
- Potassium: 309 mg
- Cholesterol: 13 mg
- Vitamin A: 0%
- Vitamin B6: 5%
- Vitamin C: 1%
- Vitamin D: 0%
- Cobalamin: 5%
- Calcium: 18%
- Magnesium: 14%
- Iron: 5%

CHICKEN EGG

Nutritional Value (in 100g) and % Daily Value*

- Calories 155
- Total Fat 11 g 16%
- Saturated fat 3.3 g 16%
- Polyunsaturated fat 1.4 g

- Monounsaturated fat 4.1 g
- Cholesterol 373 mg 124%
- Sodium 124 mg 5%
- Potassium 126 mg 3%
- Total Carbohydrate 1.1 g 0%
- Dietary fiber 0 g 0%
- Sugar 1.1 g
- Protein 13 g 26%
- Vitamin A 10%
- Vitamin C 0%
- Calcium 5%
- Iron 6%
- Vitamin D 21%
- Vitamin B-6 5%
- Cobalamin 18%
- Magnesium 2%

TURKEY

Nutritional Value (in 100g) and % Daily Value*

- Calories: 189
- Total Fat: 7 g
- Polyunsaturated fat 2.1 g
- Monounsaturated fat 2.6 g
- Trans fat 0.1 g
- Cholesterol 109 mg 36%
- Sodium 103 mg 4%
- Potassium 239 mg 6%
- Total Carbohydrate 0.1 g 0%
- Dietary fiber 0 g 0%
- Sugar 0 g
- Protein 29 g 58%
- Vitamin A 0%
- Vitamin C 0%

- Calcium 1%
- Iron 6%
- Vitamin D 3%
- Vitamin B-6 30%
- Cobalamin 16%
- Magnesium

GOOSE

Nutritional Value (in 100g)

- Protein (g) 20.66
- Fat (g) 3.42
- Total saturated fat (g) 0.52
- Total Mono-unsaturated fat (g) 0.69
- Total Poly-unsaturated fat (g) 0.30
- Cholesterol (mg) 68
- Calcium (mg) 3
- Iron (mg) 5.02
- Magnesium (mg) 25
- Phosphorus (mg) 218
- Potassium (mg) 286
- Sodium (mg) 42
- Zinc (mg) 1.43
- Selenium (mg) N/A
- Vitamin C (mg) 0.0
- Thiamin (mg) 0.24
- Riboflavin 1.30
- Niacin (mg) 5.58
- Vitamin A (IU) 32
- Total Folate (mcg)

GOOSE EGG

Nutritional Value (in 100g) and % Daily Value*

- Calories 185
- Total Fat 13 g 20%
- Saturated fat 3.6 g 18%
- Polyunsaturated fat 1.7 g
- Monounsaturated fat 6 g
- Cholesterol 852 mg 284%
- Sodium 138 mg 5%
- Potassium 210 mg 6%
- Total Carbohydrate 1.4 g 0%
- Dietary fiber 0 g 0%
- Sugar 0.9 g
- Protein 14 g 28%
- Vitamin A 13%
- Vitamin C 0%
- Calcium 6%
- Iron 19%
- Vitamin D 16%
- Vitamin B-6 10%
- Cobalamin 85%
- Magnesium 4%

RABBIT

Nutritional Value (in 100g)

- Calories: 173 calories
- Protein: 33 g
- Fat: 3.5 g
- Saturated fat: 1.1 g
- Monounsaturated fat: 1 g
- Polyunsaturated fat: 0.7 g
- Carbohydrate: 0 g
- Sodium: 45 mg
- Cholesterol: 123 mg
- potassium: 343 mg

DEER

Nutritional Value (in 100g) and % Daily Value*

- Calories 158
- Total Fat 3.2 g 4%
- Saturated fat 1.3 g 6%
- Polyunsaturated fat 0.6 g
- Monounsaturated fat 0.9 g
- Cholesterol 112 mg 37%
- Sodium 54 mg 2%
- Potassium 335 mg 9%
- Total Carbohydrate 0 g 0%
- Dietary fiber 0 g 0%
- Protein 30 g 60%
- Vitamin A 0%
- Vitamin C 0%
- Calcium 0%
- Iron 25%
- Vitamin D 0%
- Vitamin B-6 0%
- Cobalamin 0%
- Magnesium 6%

TUNA

Nutritional Value (in 100g)

- Total calories: 130
- Calories from fat: 5.3
- Total fat: 0.6g
- Cholesterol: 47 mg
- Protein: 29 g
- Carbohydrate: 0 g
- Potassium: 527 mg
- Sodium: 54 mg

MACKEREL

Nutritional Value (in 100g) and % Daily Value*

- Total Calories: 305
- Protein: 19 g
- Total fat: 25 g (38% of the total nutritional content of Mackerel)
- Saturated fat: 7 g
- Polyunsaturated: 6 g
- Monounsaturated fat: 8 g
- Carbohydrates: 0 g
- Potassium: 520 mg
- Cholesterol: 95 mg
- Sodium: 4 450 mg
- Vitamin A: 3%
- Vitamin B 6: 20%
- Vitamin C: 0%
- Vitamin D: 251%
- Calcium: 6%
- Cobalamin: 200%
- Iron: 7%
- Magnesium: 15%

SALMON

Nutritional Value (in 100g) and % Daily Value*

- Total Fat: 14g
- Polyunsaturated fat: 3 g
- Monounsaturated fat: 5 g
- Saturated: 3 8 g
- Cholesterol: 88 mg
- Protein: 27 g
- Carbohydrate: 0
- Vitamin A: 3%

- Vitamin B 6: 200%
- Vitamin C: 0 %
- Vitamin D: 0%
- Calcium: 1%
- Cobalamin: 5%
- Iron: 7%
- Magnesium: 5%

CAT FISH

Nutritional Value (in 100g) and % Daily Value*

- Calories: 129
- Protein: 16 g
- Fat: 7 g
- Saturated: 2 g
- Monounsaturated: 4 g
- Polyunsaturated: 1 g
- Carbohydrate: 0 g
- Sugar: 0 g
- Fiber: 0 g
- Thiamin
  - Amount: .4 mg
  - Daily Value: 24%
- Niacin
  - Amount: 2.1 mg
  - Daily Value: 11%
- Vitamin B12
- Amount: 2.4 mcg
- Daily Value: 40%
- Phosphorus
- Amount: 208 mg
- Daily Value: 21%
- Selenium
- Amount: 12.3 mcg

CRAB

Nutritional Value (in 100g) and % Daily Value*

- Calories 84
- Total Fat 0.6g 1 %
- Saturated Fat 0.1g 0 %
- Cholesterol 42mg 14 %
- Sodium 836mg 36 %
- Total Carbohydrate 0g 0 %
- Dietary Fiber 0g 0 %
- Protein 18g 36 %
- Vitamin D mcg N/A
- Calcium 46.00mg 4 %
- Iron 0.59mg 3 %
- Potassium 204mg 4 %

PRAWN

Nutritional Value (in 100g) and % Daily Value*

- Calories 119
- 3%Total Fat 1.7g grams
- 3% Saturated Fat 0.5g grams
- Trans Fat 0g grams
- Polyunsaturated Fat 0.6g grams
- Monounsaturated Fat 0.4g grams
- 70%Cholesterol 211mg milligrams
- 39%Sodium 947mg milligrams
- 5%Potassium 170mg milligrams
- 1%Total Carbohydrates 1.5g grams
- 0% Dietary Fiber 0g grams
- Sugars 0g grams
- Protein 23g grams

- 6% Vitamin A
- 0% Vitamin C
- 7% Calcium
- 1.8% Iron

KANGAROO

Nutritional Value (in 100g) and % Daily Value*

- Calories from Fat 30
- Calories 125
- 5%Total Fat 3.4g grams
- 6% Saturated Fat 1.2g grams
- Trans Fat 0g grams
- 21%Cholesterol 62mg milligrams
- 2%Sodium 48mg milligrams
- 10%Potassium 356mg milligrams
- 0%Total Carbohydrates 0g grams
- 0% Dietary Fiber 0g grams
- Sugars 0g grams
- Protein 22g grams
- 0% Vitamin A
- 0% Vitamin C
- 1% Calcium
- 5% Iron

DOG

As other meats, dog meat is the flesh and other edible parts derived from dogs which historically has been recorded that human consumption of dog meat is in every part of the world; commonly consumed as of the 21st century in countries like China, India, South Korea, Vietnam, Nigeria, Switzerland, etc.

In 2014, it was statistically documented that 25 million dogs are eaten each year by humans worldwide.

In some climes, their culture considers the consumption of dog meat as part of their custom or for a day-to-day cuisine whiles other cultures views it as a taboo. The different cultural stance doesn't allow this conversation about the ethics of eating dog meat to be had without nuance, you cannot categorically disregard another culture because you do not understand it.

Nutritional Value (in 100g)

- Protein: 19 g
- Total Fat: 20.2g
- Carbohydrate: 0.1 g

How To SUCCEED ON THE CARNIVoRE DIET

It is important to start the diet well in order to help prevent and also overcome the side effects that the diet may bring in the first days or weeks. Since almost everyone is used to carbohydrates, our bodies may react badly or rebel when carbohydrate sources are suddenly eliminated from the diet.

PLAN YoUR MEALS AHEAD

Below are some examples of meals that serve as menu ideas for a beginner in the carnivore diet.

Day 1

- Breakfast: steak with grass fed butter
- Lunch: Salmon or mackerel or catfish with water
- Dinner: Eggs and water
- Snacks:
    - Chicken salad
    - Beef jockey

Day 2

- Breakfast: Roasted liver and gizzard
- Lunch: steak and water
- Dinner: roasted fatty fish with lard or tallow
- Snacks:
    - Chicken salad
    - Beef jockey

Other meals to try:

- Bacon and goose egg
- Steak and chicken egg
- Pork and duck egg

- Mackerel
- Tuna
- Salmon
- Chicken salad
- Lungs and eggs

Looking for more recipes? At the end of this book you will find a cookbook that includes 45 easy and delicious meat-based, non-strict carnivore diet recipes to start your meal plan. You'll find recipes for every type of meat: red meat, white meat, seafood, organ meat. Have fun cooking and enjoy your diet.

EAT UNTIL YoU ARE FULL

The main rule to follow is to eat until you feel full. Your appetite will change over the course of the first month. Don't go hungry and eat as much as you want: your body needs energy and you have to provide it. Go for fatty cuts of meat and don't limit yourself to lean cuts. The saturated and unsaturated animal fats found in meat provide your body with additional essential nutrients it needs daily to stay healthy, along with the proteins, minerals, vitamins and other nutrients you get from the lean parts of meat. Plus, adding fat makes any food tastier, so it's a win-win for everyone.

ASSUME ENoUGH FAT

Get adequate amounts of animal fats along with meat consumption. The basis of this diet is to eat a lot of fat to allow the body to enter ketosis, a metabolic state that facilitates weight loss. The high protein nature of this diet means that when a lot of fats are consumed, they are used for energy instead of proteins, as in the case of gluconeogenesis.

DRINK LoTS OF WATER

Choosing to drink only water depends on how strict you want to be in your way of following the carnivore diet. Most people recommend trying to drink water only for the first 30 days. Try adding a little salt to your water for extra electrolytes. A complete or strict follower will eat only meat and drink only water. Some long-term carnivore diet followers may find that they still wish to drink coffee or tea. This is allowed as long as no sugar or sweeteners are added to hot drinks. Avoid hot or cold drinks with added carbohydrates such as: sodas, plant drinks, energy drinks, etc.

EXERCISE REGULARLY

While on this diet, take a lot of exercise. It is very important to engage in physical activity as health experts have found out that lack of physical activity or a sedentary lifestyle is a potential risk for developing obesity, type 2 diabetes, cardiovascular diseases and other non-communicable diseases. It is very important to be physically active.

TRY INTERMITTENT FASTING

Intermittent fasting is a smart way to reduce or stop your calorie intake in order to facilitate weight loss. The carnivore diet works very well in combination with intermittent fasting because the meat diet is super satiating and can facilitate intermittent fasting by helping you not even feel hungry.

AVoID SUPPLEMENTS

You should only use supplements when you can no longer make progress in building muscle mass. This should happen at around 6, 9 or 12 months. When it comes to achieving good health or achieving the goals most people set on a diet, supplements do more harm than good. Bodybuilding can be an exception. Carrying a lot of muscles around isn't something the body "wants" to do. Muscle is energy expensive to maintain.

HOw TO SAVE MONEY ON THE CARNIVORE DIET

CALCULATE YOUR EXISTING FOOD BUDGET

Before you head out add up the costs of all the non-meat and non-dairy stuff you buy. Now you have a baseline to aim for and try to get all your carnivore food planned out for the week with that total budget in mind.

WORK OUT YOUR EXACT MEAT INTAKE

Based on the average energy need per day of 2000 calories, you can start creating a carnivore diet meal plan. If you're a bodybuilder in a bulking phase, then you may need to add 10% to 20%, and if you've got some weight loss goals, then you want to reduce it by at least 10%. Now, the average cut of beef, chicken, and pork will have about 600 calories per pound, but you can stretch that to 800 calories by going for ones with more fat.

CHOOSE GROUND BEEF INSTEAD OF STEAK

Steak and in-particular grass-fed steak can be pretty expensive. While ground beef might not be as nutritionally rich as steak, that's not to say it doesn't have its benefits, and being cheaper is one of these.

GET FAT TRIMMINGS

Fattier cuts of ground beef are going to be cheaper and have more calories than lean cuts. You can add fat trimmings to your burgers and steaks to increase the fat ratio which in turn makes you more satiated. Just go to the local butcher and ask them for some. Sometimes they will give them to you for free and other times you may have to pay for them but they are cheap, like 50 cents a pound cheap.

LOOK OUT FOR SALES

You can really score some deals at your conventional grocery store: if a certain meat isn't selling they will slap on the reduced price sales stickers. The meat that is about to expire in a day will have tremendous reductions in price, like 25-75 percent off.

You can also ask the butcher manager when they usually markdown about to expire meats. So when you see the major markdowns and sales, go ahead and stock up and put what you're not going to use that week in the freezer.

BUY DIRECTLY FROM A FARM

Going directly through a farm can save you tons of money on beef, eggs, chicken, pork, and even more exotic meats.

BUY IN BULK

If you can buy in bulk, you can save a ton of money. Buying in bulk can be more difficult for some than others, for example due to limited freezer space, or a temporary living situation. Look out for grass-fed and pasture-raised farms near you, or try buying in-bulk online looking for sales. When you buy a whole cow, you'll get organ meats, tons of steak, and lots of other goodies, and save tons of money in the process.

TRY INTERMITTENT FASTING

Last but not least, intermittent fasting is a great way to both lose weight and, of course, spend less on meat.

How To BUILD MUSCLE ON THE CARNIVoRE DIET

CARNIVoRE DIET AND MUSCLE BUILDING

The carnivore diet only allows you to eat animal products. Meat and eggs are the staples of the carnivore diet. The bulk of food comes from animal flesh like beef, bison, chicken and fish. Dairy is also allowed in some cases. Vegetables, grains, rice and fruits cannot be eaten.

For this reason, the carnivore diet is a controversial topic because it challenges conventional nutrition doctrine. Some say that eating only meat is unhealthy and leads to illness and disease. Others say that eating meat puts you on the fast track to a heart attack. Make sure you eat enough fat on the carnivore diet. There's a reason steaks have fat on them naturally: you need enough fat to help digest protein. As a thriving carnivore, your chronic systemic inflammation will subside by the day.

The number one ingredient for muscle building is a specific set of amino acids that are the building blocks of protein. It would not be uncommon for bodybuilders to aim for 1 to 1.5 grams of protein per pound of body weight. That's a lot of meat to digest, and something many performance athletes take a long time to get used to.

No matter what your body composition is or what you're aiming for, you cannot achieve a lot of muscle building and fat loss without certain minerals and vitamins. They're vital for your immune system and overall health, but so many other processes are also reliant on them. In fact B, C and D vitamins are the most crucial when it comes to healthy muscle growth, especially B12. Therefore, do not neglect nutrients while on the diet.

Zinc, magnesium, and iron are three of the essential minerals that your body needs when it comes to supporting muscle growth. Zinc is vital for testosterone production, while magnesium helps to produce energy and aids in muscle recovery. That leaves iron, which is a critical mineral to increase red blood cell count that delivers the oxygen to muscle fibers. People who follow the carnivore diet, or other high-fat diets, often claim that it can increase testosterone levels. And this, in turn, can lead to a number of benefits ranging from fat loss to muscle gain, increased libido, greater energy and endurance, and more.

When you plan a diet to gain muscle weight, you will need to watch the amount of calories you consume. The average healthy adult will require about 2000 calories a day, but during a bulking phase that kind of intake will need to increase significantly. There is no one best meat for bodybuilding, it's important to know your body. But one thing to avoid is the very lean cuts that have little to no fat. On the meat-only diet, you will need all the energy from fat to fuel your strength training. Aim for lots of beef and chicken as it provides a great combination of fat and protein and add in some fish.

There are a lot of ways of training to build muscle. Strength training, Olympic lifting, cross fit and so on all work. They all can build muscle. But they all can give different results as well. People tend to adapt quite quickly to strength training because it mainly uses the creatine-phosphate energy system.

For one, you need to become fat adapted. Becoming fat adapted essentially means your body can utilize fat as a source of fuel in the most efficient way possible. This is important for someone who wants to undertake any kind of exercise program because it's the difference between poor performance and great progress. You'll know when you've become fat adapted because you'll be able to go for long periods of time between meals without feeling hungry. You'll know you're fat adapted for workouts when you begin to return to exceed your previous personal bests.

For most people, training will suffer on the carnivore diet, especially for those who spend most of time doing glucose specific training like strength training or bodybuilding. Although muscle size and quality often increase with no training at all when starting out on the carnivore diet due to the increased protein intake, it's not without its challenges.

Strength training while on the carnivore diet is a minefield of information because we hardly have any reputable research on the topic. One of the biggest myths about strength training is that you need lots of carbs to lift heavy.

While this may be true as you go through the fat adaption phase, most seasoned low carb strong men always return to or exceed their previous personal bests, when you consider strength to weight ratio. In other words, strength athletes will almost certainly get smaller in size due to the fat loss and lack of water retention, but muscle mass will increase due to the extra protein intake.

6 TIPS To BUILD MUSCLE ON THE CARNIVoRE DIET

1. **Find your daily baseline.** You should have a feel for how much you eat on a daily basis. Once adapted to the carnivore diet, appetite regulates by itself. Find your daily "normal." You should have a good feel for how much this is. Let's say, for example, you eat 3lbs of meat per day. And this meat consists mainly fatty cuts. Also if you eat foods such as cheese for example, know how much on average. The whole point is to know what your daily average consumption is.
2. **Exceed your baseline.** Once you know your basic food consumption, you want to increase it. Add a little more

food. Crucial: This food you add must contain protein. Don't just add butter. Add the meat. Add the eggs. It doesn't have to be in a significant amount. Don't worry about counting and add some protein food on top of your baseline.

3. **Increase progressively.** Then every month, or every 6 weeks or whatever you feel is a good pace, increase consumption again. How many weeks you go in between increases is not as important as the idea of progression. Continue this month after month (regularly). Keep in mind that progression is not going to be easy. You will be too full to continue to progressively eat more. Plus a big jump like this will likely result in more fat gain than you want. Then you have to eat to maintain body fat levels, plus the extra on top of that to fuel new muscle growth. Slow progression is the key.

4. **Take supplements.** Supplements should only come into play when you can no longer progress. This should happen at around 6, 9 or 12 months. When it comes to achieving most people's health goals, supplements do more harm than good. Bodybuilding can be an exception. Carrying a lot of muscles around isn't something the body "wants" to do. Muscle is energy expensive to maintain.

5. **Add whey protein.** When you reach a stage of not being to take in any more, add whey protein to increase total consumption without getting overly full.

6. **Add more protein.** If you added in whey for several months and need to increase consumption further, and you can't do it with more whole food, then I'd try adding in some more protein powder. The collagen will provide a more diverse amino acid profile while the whey keeps a high concentration of branched chain amino acids.

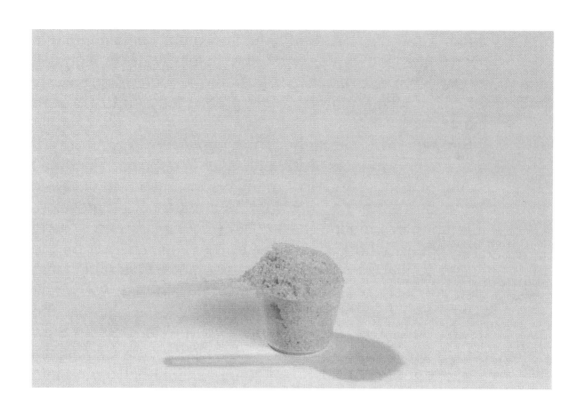

FREQUENTLY ASKED QUESTIONS

IS THE CARNIVORE DIET HEALTHY?

Answer: The carnivore diet is healthy when done properly. The diet of carnivores is very restrictive and does not allow the intake of plants that can cause allergies or the intake of foods that are high in carbohydrates or foods that give empty calories. The empty calories come from foods or beverages which mainly include sugar, fats and oils, and also drinks which are mainly alcohols. Intake of empty calories could be a cause of weight gain and also a precursor to the onset of type 2 diabetes. Since the carnivore diet restricts all of these foods, the diet does not give space or give the potential for diseases resulting from the intake of plants and empty calories. Thus, we can say that the carnivore diet is healthy.

IS THIS DIET GOOD FOR MY HEART HEALTH?

Answer: This is a very controversial issue because some people have been proven to have a better heart health while on the carnivore diet, while some studies show that eating too much red meat is bad for the heart. This is because meat has the potential of being high in cholesterol and also in saturated fat. Saturated fat is bad because it raises the Low Density Lipo proteins which are the bad cholesterol in the body. This can lead to increased risk of heart diseases. However, it is noteworthy that the studies being carried out include people who have other behavioral lifestyles that could increase the risk of developing heart disease, such as smoking and alcohol consumption, so we cannot conclude that being on the carnivore diet alone can lead to heart diseases.

CAN I REALLY LOSE WEIGHT ON THE CARNIVORE DIET?

Answer: The carnivore diet actually helps you lose weight. This is because it is very high in protein and very low in carbohydrates. A diet of this type leads to a low level of carbohydrates in the body, which is at the base of weight loss. Since protein is very filling, the amount of calories consumed in a protein food meal (in this case, meat) will be much lower than the amount of calories consumed in a carbohydrate meal. This helps the body lose weight, because the calorie intake is not enough to accumulate body fat. Also, if you eat high-fat meats, your body may well be in ketosis, a state where fat is used as a fuel source for the body, thus greatly reducing the fat stored as body fat and this in turn leads to weight loss.

CAN I REALLY HEAL FROM FOOD ALLERGIES AND AUTOIMMUNITY WHILE ON THIS DIET?

Answer: Foods from plant sources have been held culprit as the main cause of food allergy and also autoimmunity. Food allergy occurs when the proteins present in food are interpreted incorrectly by the immune system to be poisons. Autoimmunity is a condition in which the immune system fights against its own healthy cells as though they are foreign invaders. This leads to a large number of diseases called autoimmune diseases. The compounds that cause food allergy and autoimmunity (majorly Lectins and gluten) are mainly found in plant sources of food (e.g. wheat, peanut and soybean). So eating an all meat diet as in the carnivore diet really helps circumvent the possibility of being exposed to those compounds that cause food allergy and also autoimmunity.

CAN ONE'S MUSCLE MASS INCREASE WHILE ON THIS DIET?

Answer: Since this diet is high in protein and protein is the nutrient needed for tissue building, muscle mass can increase during this diet. It is important to note that it is muscle mass (not fat tissue) that has the potential for growth during this diet.

IS THE CARNIVORE DIET BETTER THAN THE KETO DIET?

Answer. There is no real answer to if the carnivore diet is better than the keto diet because each of them have their peculiarities. Both diets are used in shedding weight however through different mechanisms: the carnivore diet is high in protein while the keto diet is high in fat. Asides from helping to shed weight, both diets also have their other specific advantages. This is why it cannot be concluded that one diet is absolutely better than the other.

IS THE CARNIVORE DIET ACTUALLY EXPENSIVE?

Answer. the carnivore diet isn't exactly expensive since you won't be eating much meat anyway because of the satiety effect. Actually, considering that all you need to buy is just meat, eggs and water, it's not expensive compared to when you had to buy groceries and meat and water. So to be on the carnivore diet is not actually expensive.

WHAT ARE THE FOODS ALLOWED ON THE CARNIVORE DIET?

Answer. The foods allowed on the carnivore diet are meat (lamb, beef, bacon, ham, pork, rabbit, turkey, chicken, duck etc.), organ meat (liver, kidney, heart, brain, gizzard etc.), fish (sardine, salmon, titus, lobster, cat fish, herring, mackerel), crab, egg (chicken, turkey, duck) and sometimes dairy.

WHAT FOODS SHOULD I AVOID WHILE ON THIS DIET?

Answer. Avoid any food that is not from animal sources: vegetables, grains, legumes, fruits, tubers, potatoes, bananas, vegetable oil, chocolate and even meats that have been already processed.

CAN I INCLUDE DAIRY IN A CARNIVORE DIET?

Answer. if you don't have an existing allergy to dairy products, they can be included in the carnivore diet.

CAN I USE SPICES IN COOKING MY MEAT?

Answer. spices that do not contain any amount of carbohydrates and sugar are allowed, but in moderate quantity. Examples of spices that are allowed are salt, pepper and herbs. However on a very strict carnivore diet, use animal based fats, lard and tallow to cook your meals.

CAN I DRINK TEA ON THE CARNIVORE DIET?

Answer. No. Tea and also coffee are discouraged on the carnivore diet. This is because tea and coffee are from plant sources and might contain a significant amount of sugar or carbohydrate.

CAN I USE NUTRIENT SUPPLEMENTS WHILE ON THE DIET?

Answer. If you work out or you're concerned that you are not eating enough nutrients, you can take nutrient supplements in a carnivore diet plan. However, it might supply the body with nutrients that are not needed while on the carnivore diet and defeat the purpose of being on the diet.

ARE SNACKS ALLOWED?

Answer: Yes, certain snacks are allowed while on the carnivore diet. Snacks include tuna, snacks made from beacon, meat jerkies, meat bites, salami snacks, chicken salad, liver salad, salmon, crab, sushi.

HOW MUCH MEAT DO I ACTUALLY NEED TO EAT?

Answer: the amount of meat you can eat on this diet is the amount of meat you can eat till you're full.

HOW MANY MEALS PER DAY DO I NEED TO EAT WHILE ON THE CARNIVORE DIET?

Answer: while on this diet, you can eat as many meals as you want. This is because it is a low-carb diet, so the calories in a meal are not many. Also, because protein is filling, you would most likely end up eating no more than your body needs in a day.

HOW DO I GET ENERGY WHILE I'M ON THE CARNIVORE DIET?

Answer: Energy is obtained from a process called gluconeogenesis in which protein molecules are converted into glucose for energy. It is the synthesis of new glucose in the body. Gluconeogenesis helps supply the body with glucose obtained from proteins to fuel the metabolic activities that take place in the body.

HOW WILL I GET A SUPPLY OF VITAMINS AND MINERALS WHILE ON THIS DIET?

Answer: If you eat different types of meat and include eggs and dairy products, you should get adequate amounts of the nutrients your body needs.

IS THERE EVIDENCE FOR THE CARNIVORE DIET?

Answer: There is fossil evidence showing that some of the earliest groups of people were carnivores. There is also some scientific research evidence supporting the carnivore diet. However, not much research has been done on it.

CAN ONE REALLY SURVIVE ON MEAT ALONE?

Answer: There are many claims that some of our ancestors only survived on meat, such as the Inuit population in Canada. Mikalia Peterson and her father (the people who brought the carnivore diet to the fore), also claimed to be on a diet alone and survived and also had greater benefits than when they were on a high-carb diet.

In addition, meat contains minerals such as iron and zinc, it also contains some of the B complex vitamins in addition to proteins and fats. Since the egg is still a product of animal origin, it is allowed in the diet of carnivores. Egg contains many vitamins and minerals that are essential for life. So, if the egg is included in the carnivore diet, surely this is more complete. Also, since the diet is very filling (due to its high level of protein and fat), it doesn't leave you hungry, so you can actually survive on the diet.

HOW LONG DOES IT TAKE BEFORE I GET USED TO THIS DIET?

Answer: The ability to adapt to a new diet varies from person to person. The factors responsible for the difference are genetics, previous diet, environment and the type of new diet. It takes an average of a month to get used to the carnivore diet, especially if you ate mostly carbohydrates before starting the carnivore diet. The body needs time to get used to having to draw energy from proteins and fats. So, on average, in a month your body should be accustomed to the carnivore diet.

CAN I BE ON THIS DIET FOR A LONG TIME?

Answer: You can follow this diet for a long time. However, it is advisable not to follow the diet for more than 8 months. This is because the body actually needs both animal and plant sources to be healthy. Since in the carnivore diet, due to its highly restrictive nature, there is an undoubted food monotony (lack of diversified food) that could lead to completely losing interest in eating. This can lead to anorexia, resulting in negative health effects, so it is not recommended to follow the carnivore diet for a long time. Once you have reached the reason or reasons for starting the diet (e.g. losing weight, having a clearer mind, controlling autoimmune diseases, controlling digestive problems or improving cognitive function), it is advisable to stop the diet and return to a more varied and balanced diet between animal and vegetable sources.

CARNIVORE COOKBOOK

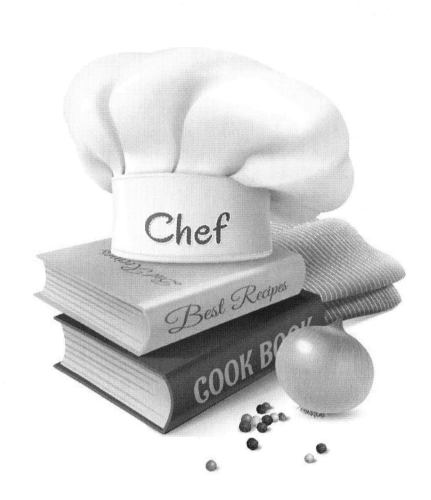

RED MEAT RECIPES

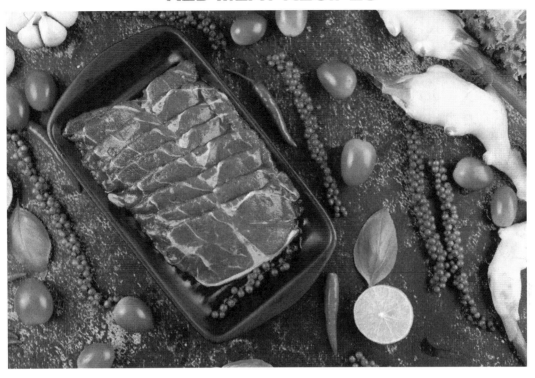

BACON APPLE CHICKEN

Nutritional value

Amount per serving.

- Calories 486
- % Daily Value*
- Total Fat 18.2g 28%
- Saturated Fat 9.2g 46%
- Trans Fat 0g
- Cholesterol 0mg 0%
- Sodium 1,600mg 67%
- Potassium 0mg 0%
- Total Carbohydrate 47g 16%
- Dietary Fiber 3.6g 14%
- Sugars 3.9g
- Protein 31.7g 63%
- Vitamin A 0%
- Vitamin C 0%
- Calcium 0%
- Iron 0%

Percent Daily Values are based on a 2,000 calorie diet. Your daily values may be higher or lower depending on your calorie needs.

Ingredients

- 4 chicken breasts
- 8 slices of bacon
- 1 teaspoon of garlic powder
- 1 cup of barbeque sauce

Method of preparation

Wrap each piece of chicken in 2 pieces of bacon and place in the bottom of a slow cooker. Sprinkle with garlic powder. Mix the barbecue sauce and pour over the chicken. Cook on low heat for about 6-8 hours until completely cooked.

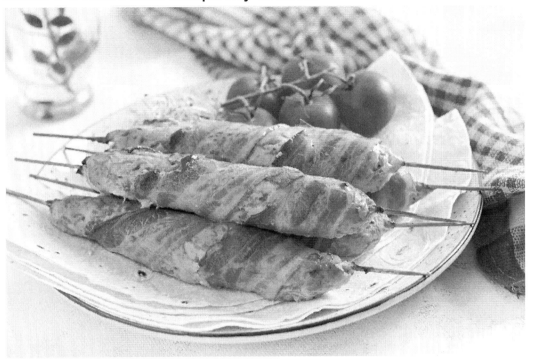

BACON MEATBALLS

Nutritional value

Amount per serving.

- Calories: 163
- % Daily Values*
- Total Fat: 14.2g 22%
- Saturated Fat 5.506g 28%
- Polyunsaturated Fat 0.313g
- Monounsaturated Fat 5.114g
- Cholesterol 51mg 17%
- Sodium 260mg 11%
- Total Carbohydrate 0.11g 0%
- Dietary Fiber 0g 0%
- Sugars 0.03g
- Protein 7.64g
- Calcium 330mg 33%
- Iron 8.10mg 45%
- Potassium 87mg 2%
- Vitamin A 1000IU 20%
- Vitamin C 0mg 0%

The % Daily Value (DV) tells you how much a nutrient in a serving of food contributes to a daily diet. 2,000 calories a day is used for general nutrition advice.

Ingredients

- 6 slices of bacon
- ½ of an onion
- 1 ½ pounds of ground beef
- 1 large egg
- 2 tablespoons of mustard
- 3 cloves of garlic

- 1 tablespoon of Worcestershire sauce
- Some salt and freshly grounded pepper
- 2 tablespoons of vegetable oil

Method of preparation

Put the onion and bacon into a food processor until finely chopped. Then transfer it into a bowl and add beef, parsley, almond meal, egg, garlic, mustard, Worcestershire sauce, ¾ teaspoon of salt and ½ teaspoon of pepper and mix until just combined. Dampen your hands and begin to form the meatballs. Heat the vegetable oil in a large non-stick pan over medium heat. Add the meatballs in and cook, until browned and cooked through add the sauce to the meatballs and continue to cook over medium heat until the sauce is simmering and the meatballs are heated through, about 2 minutes.

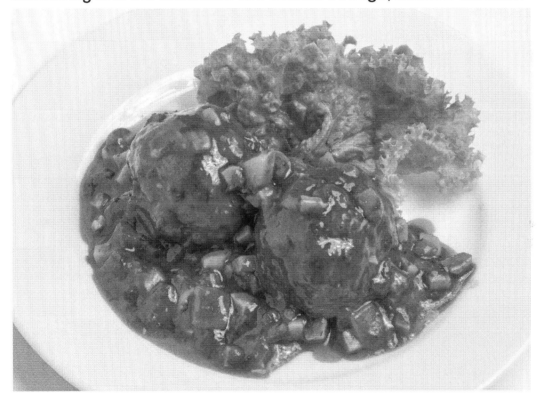

BEEF BRISKET

Nutritional value

Amount per 100 grams.

- Calories 155
- % Daily Value*
- Total Fat 7 g 10%
- Saturated fat 2.6 g 13%
- Polyunsaturated fat 0.2 g
- Monounsaturated fat 3.5 g
- Cholesterol 62 mg 20%
- Sodium 79 mg 3%
- Potassium 330 mg 9%
- Total Carbohydrate 0 g 0%
- Dietary fiber 0 g 0%
- Sugar 0 g
- Protein 21 g 42%
- Vitamin A 0%
- Vitamin C 0%
- Calcium 0%
- Iron 10%
- Vitamin D 0%
- Vitamin B-6 20%
- Cobalamin 40%
- Magnesium 5%

*Per cent Daily Values are based on a 2,000 calorie diet.

Ingredients

- 3- 4 pounds of a brisket cut of bee
- ¾ cup of barbeque sauce
- ¼ cup soy sauce
- 1 cup of water

Method of preparation

Preheat oven to 300ºF, in a bowl, mix together the barbecue sauce, soy sauce, and water. Place a large piece of aluminum foil in a roasting pan. Add the brisket and spread the barbeque sauce mixture generously over meat. Wrap the brisket in the aluminum foil so it's well sealed, like a package. Bake for 3 hours for a 3 pound roast and 1 more hour for every additional pound of meat.

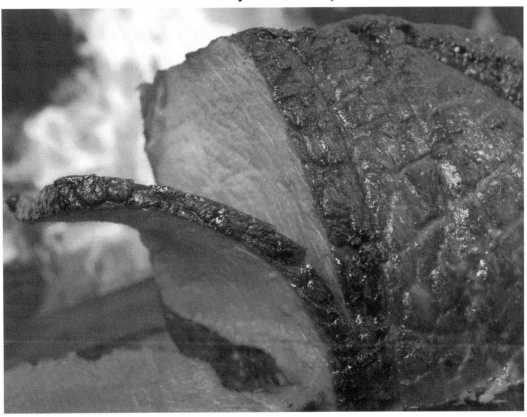

BRAISED BEEF

Nutritional value

Amount per 100 grams.

- Calories 471
- % Daily Value*
- Total Fat 42 g 64%
- Saturated fat 18 g 90%
- Polyunsaturated fat 1.5 g
- Monounsaturated fat 19 g
- Cholesterol 94 mg 31%
- Sodium 50 mg 2%
- Potassium 224 mg 6%
- Total Carbohydrate 0 g 0%
- Dietary fiber 0 g 0%
- Sugar 0 g
- Protein 22 g 44%
- Vitamin A 0%
- Vitamin C 0%
- Calcium 1%
- Iron 12%
- Vitamin D 6%
- Vitamin B-6 10%
- Cobalamin 43%
- Magnesium 3%

*Per cent Daily Values are based on a 2,000 calorie diet. Your daily values may be higher or lower depending on your calorie needs.

Ingredients

- 3 or 3 ½ boneless beef chunk
- 6 tablespoons of olive oil
- 1 tablespoon of cumin

- 1 tablespoon of paprika
- 2 tablespoons of salt
- 1 tablespoon of black pepper
- 1 large onion
- 2 garlic cloves
- ¾ cup of red wine
- ¼ cup of water

Method of preparation

Cut the beef into large chunks and heat olive oil in a pot over high heat. Remove when brown and set aside. Cook the onions in the same pot until they are fully cooked (translucent). In an oven pan begin layering the ingredients in the following order; ½ teaspoon of cumin, 1/2 teaspoon of paprika, 1 teaspoon of salt, 1/2 teaspoon of black pepper, ½ sautéed onion and ½ garlic (preferably blended) add the red wine and water and place the lid on top. Place the pot unto the stove and bring it to boil then place the pot in the oven for 1 ½ or 2 hours at around 180 degrees Celsius. Leave until fully cooked.

BRANDIED HAM

Nutritional value

Amount per serving.

- Calories 194.5
- Total Fat 9.2 g
- Saturated Fat 2.5 g
- Polyunsaturated Fat 2.5 g
- Monounsaturated Fat 3.7 g
- Cholesterol 13.8 mg
- Sodium 472.5 mg
- Potassium 828.7 mg
- Total Carbohydrate 7.7 g
- Dietary Fiber 2.6 g
- Sugars 1.2 g
- Protein 21.2 g
- Vitamin A 22.1 %
- Vitamin B-12 8.9 %
- Vitamin B-6 11.4 %
- Vitamin C 26.3 %
- Vitamin D 3.3 %
- Vitamin E 15.0 %
- Calcium 10.9 %
- Copper 14.3 %
- Folate 38.1 %
- Iron 22.4 %
- Magnesium 9.3 %
- Manganese 17.2 %
- Niacin 13.5 %
- Pantothenic Acid 39.5 %
- Phosphorus 27.0 %
- Riboflavin 37.3 %

- Selenium 53.9 %
- Thiamin 28.9 %
- Zinc 17.0 %

*Percent Daily Values are based on a 2,000 calorie diet.

Ingredients

- 1 ½ cups packed dark-brown sugar
- ¼ cup of brandy or bourbon
- 2 tablespoons of grainy mustard
- 1 bone in half ham

Method of preparation

In a small saucepan, combine sugar, brandy, and mustard. Bring to a boil in a pot and cook until glaze is thick and syrupy for about 3 minutes. Preheat oven to 275 degrees. Using a sharp knife cut off hard rind from ham (if any. Place ham, cut side down, in a roasting pan or on a baking sheet and cover tightly with foil. Brush ham generously with glaze, making sure to coat all exposed areas. Increase oven temperature to 350 degrees and bake, uncovered, until glaze is sticky and ham is browned, about 35 minutes. Serve warm or at room temperature.

BEEF IN BEER

Ingredients

- 2 tablespoons beef drippings or butter, plus more as needed
- 1 tablespoon olive oil
- 3 pounds of sirloin tip
- 3 large onions (sliced)
- 4 cloves garlic, (chopped)
- 2 tablespoons all-purpose almond ground flax meal
- 1 tablespoon brown sugar
- 1 ½ cups beef stock
- 2 cups beer
- 1 tablespoon of red-wine vinegar
- Salt and freshly ground black pepper

Method of preparation

Heat the beef drippings and oil together in a saute pan, brown the beef strips on all sides and remove from the pan. In the same pan, fry the onions until soft, for about 15 minutes, then add the garlic for 1 minute then remove. (Check if there is fat in the pan. If not, add a good tablespoon of butter and let it melt.) Add the almond ground flax meal and sugar to the pan and cook for 1 minute. Gradually whisk in the stock and bring to a boil. At this point, turn the oven on to 160 degrees Celsius Add the beer and vinegar to the boiling stock, and bring back to a boil, cooking until thickened, about 10 minutes. Remove from the heat.

BEEF PAPRIKASH

Nutritional value

Amount per serving.

- Calories 194.5
- Total Fat 9.2 g
- Saturated Fat 2.5 g
- Polyunsaturated Fat 2.5 g
- Monounsaturated Fat 3.7 g
- Cholesterol 13.8 mg
- Sodium 472.5 mg
- Potassium 828.7 mg
- Total Carbohydrate 7.7 g
- Dietary Fiber 2.6 g
- Sugars 1.2 g
- Protein 21.2 g
- Vitamin A 22.1 %
- Vitamin B-12 8.9 %
- Vitamin B-6 11.4 %
- Vitamin C 26.3 %
- Vitamin D 3.3 %
- Vitamin E 15.0 %
- Calcium 10.9 %
- Copper 14.3 %
- Folate 38.1 %
- Iron 22.4 %
- Magnesium 9.3 %
- Manganese 17.2 %
- Niacin 13.5 %
- Pantothenic Acid 39.5 %
- Phosphorus 27.0 %
- Riboflavin 37.3 %

- Selenium 53.9 %
- Thiamin 28.9 %
- Zinc 17.0 %

*Percent Daily Values are based on a 2,000 calorie diet

Ingredients

- 2 tablespoons oil of fat origin
- 1 ½ pounds boneless beef sirloin, trimmed and cut into thin strips
- ½ cup chopped onion
- ½ cup chopped bell pepper
- 1 package of beef sauce mix
- 1 cup water
- 1 tablespoon of tomato paste
- 1 teaspoon of paprika
- 1 cup sour cream

Method of preparation

Heat the oil of fat origin in large skillet on medium-high heat. Add beef, onion and bell pepper; cook and stir 5 minutes or until beef no longer pink.

Stir in Sauce Mix, water, tomato paste and paprika until well blended.

Bring to boil. Cover. Reduce heat and simmer 10 minutes, stirring occasionally. Remove from heat Stir in sour cream

GARLIC ROSEMARY PORK CHOPS

Nutritional value

Amount per serving.

- Calories 143
- % Daily Value*
- Total Fat 3.5 g 5%
- Saturated fat 1.2 g 6%
- Polyunsaturated fat 0.5 g
- Monounsaturated fat 1.3 g
- Trans fat 0 g
- Cholesterol 73 mg 24%
- Sodium 57 mg 2%
- Potassium 421 mg 12%
- Total Carbohydrate 0 g 0%
- Dietary fiber 0 g 0%
- Sugar 0 g
- Protein 26 g 52%
- Vitamin A 0%
- Vitamin C 0%
- Calcium 0%
- Iron 6%
- Vitamin D 2%
- Vitamin B-6 35%
- Cobalamin 10%
- Magnesium 7%

*Per cent Daily Values are based on a 2,000 calorie diet.

Ingredients

- 3 lbs. of boneless pork loin, well-trimmed
- 3 cloves of minced garlic
- 2 tablespoon of grainy mustard

- 1 tablespoon of chopped rosemary
- 1 tablespoon of chopped thyme leaves
- Salt
- Freshly ground black pepper
- 3 tablespoon of melted butter
- 1 tablespoon of brown sugar

Method of preparation

Preheat oven to 400°. Line a pan with foil and place a wire rack on top. Roll the flap of the boneless loin into a cylinder and using kitchen twine, tie the pork loin every few inches. In a small bowl, mix together garlic, mustard, thyme, 1 ½ teaspoons salt, and freshly ground black pepper. Rub mixture all over pork loin and place in roasting pan fat-side down. Bake for 30 minutes. Mix melted butter and brown sugar together, and then brush on top of the pork loin. Broil for 2 minutes to let caramelize. Let it rest for 10 minutes before slicing. Serve pork warm with extra pan juices.

LAMB CHOPS

Nutritional value

Amount per serving.

- Calories: 226
- % Daily Values*
- Total Fat 17.55g 27%
- Saturated Fat 7.669g 38%
- Polyunsaturated Fat 1.302g
- Monounsaturated Fat 7.186g
- Cholesterol 68mg 23%
- Sodium 281mg 12%
- Total Carbohydrate 0g 0%
- Dietary Fiber 0g 0%
- Sugars 0g
- Protein 15.86g
- Vitamin D
- Calcium 14mg 1%
- Iron 1.40mg 8%
- Potassium 184mg 5%
- Vitamin A 0IU 0%
- Vitamin C 0mg 0%

The % Daily Value (DV) tells you how much a nutrient in a serving of food contributes to a daily diet. 2,000 calories a day is used for general nutrition advice.

Ingredients

- 4 rib lamb chops ¾ inch thick
- 1 tablespoon of oil
- Salt and freshly ground pepper

Method of preparation

Season lamb chops with salt, and pepper. Heat olive oil in a large skillet over medium heat. Add chops; cook until brown on the bottom, 4 to 5 minutes. Turn and cook until a meat thermometer reads 130 degrees (for medium-rare) and chops are evenly browned, 3 to 4 minutes more.

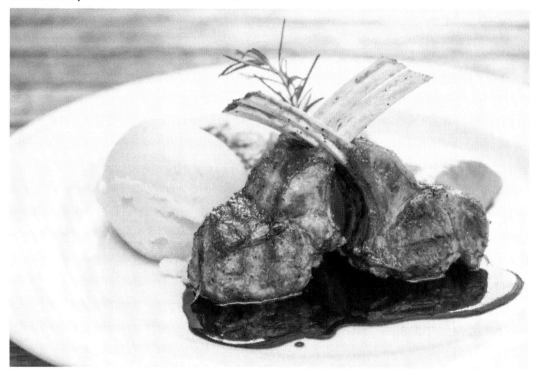

MEATLOAF

Nutritional value

Amount per 100 grams.

- Calories 149
- % Daily Value*
- Total Fat - 6 g 9%
- Saturated fat - 2.3 g 11%
- Polyunsaturated fat - 0.5 g
- Monounsaturated fat - 3 g
- Cholesterol - 46 mg 15%
- Sodium - 732 mg 30%
- Potassium 394 mg 11%
- Total Carbohydrate 4.5 g 1%
- Dietary fiber 0 g 0%
- Sugar 4.6 g
- Protein 17 g 34%
- Vitamin A 0%
- Vitamin C 0%
- Calcium 5%
- Iron 6%
- Vitamin D 8%
- Vitamin B-6 15%
- Cobalamin 33%
- Magnesium 5%

*Per cent Daily Values are based on a 2,000 calorie diet.

Ingredients

- 1 lean ground beef
- ¼ cup finely chopped onion
- 2 eggs, beaten
- 1 cup of plain bread crumbs (optional)

- 1 teaspoon of Italian seasoning
- ½ a cup of ketchup
- ½ a cup of milk

Method of preparation

Heat the oven to about 178 degrees Celsius. In a large bowl, mix the Meatloaf ingredients well. Press the mixture in an ungreased loaf pan and bake for about 40 minutes. Remove it from the oven, then spread ¼ cup of ketchup evenly over the top and bake for an additional 15 to 20 minutes. Let it cool for 10 minutes before serving.

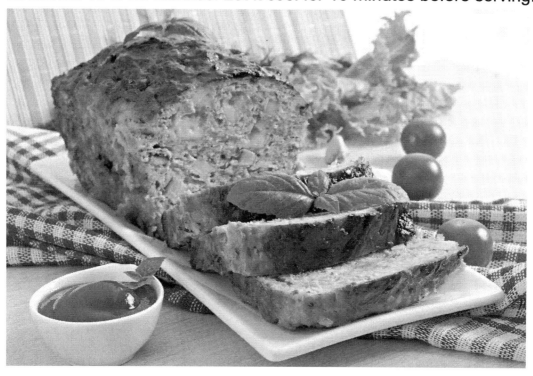

PORK TENDERLOIN

Nutritional value

Amount per serving.

- Calories 143
- % Daily Value*
- Total Fat 3.5 g 5%
- Saturated fat 1.2 g 6%
- Polyunsaturated fat 0.5 g
- Monounsaturated fat 1.3 g
- Trans fat 0 g
- Cholesterol 73 mg 24%
- Sodium 57 mg 2%
- Potassium 421 mg 12%
- Total Carbohydrate 0 g 0%
- Dietary fiber 0 g 0%
- Sugar 0 g
- Protein 26 g 52%
- Vitamin A 0%
- Vitamin C 0%
- Calcium 0%
- Iron 6%
- Vitamin D 2%
- Vitamin B-6 35%
- Cobalamin 10%
- Magnesium 7%

*Per cent Daily Values are based on a 2,000 calorie diet.

Ingredients

- 2 pounds pork tenderloin (cut into steaks)
- 2 tablespoons olive oil
- 1 tablespoon salt

- 1 teaspoon black pepper
- ¼ cup cilantro (chopped)
- ¼ teaspoon cumin
- ½ cup olive oil
- 1 tablespoon shallot (minced)
- ½ tablespoon garlic (minced)

Method of preparation

Heat the oven and pan. 10 to 20 minutes before you plan to cook, place a large cast-iron pan on the middle rack in the oven and heat the oven to 450°F. The pan will heat along with the oven. Pat the pork dry with paper towels and trim off any large pieces of surface fat. Mix any spices being used with the salt and pepper in a small bowl. Rub the spice mix onto the pork on all sides. Using oven mitts, carefully remove the hot pan from the oven. Add the oil and swirl to coat the bottom of the pan. Roast the pork for 10 minutes. Reduce the oven temperature to 400°F and continue roasting 10 to 15 minutes more then bring it out allow it to cool for 2-3 then serve.

RED BEEF CHILI

Nutritional value

Amount per serving.

- Calories 287.2
- Total Fat 12.6 g
- Saturated Fat 4.9 g
- Polyunsaturated Fat 0.9 g
- Monounsaturated Fat 5.2 g
- Cholesterol 42.4 mg
- Sodium 768.0 mg
- Potassium 490.7 mg
- Total Carbohydrate 27.7 g
- Dietary Fiber 10.5 g
- Sugars 6.3 g
- Protein 17.2 g
- Vitamin A 37.1 %
- Vitamin B-12 22.0 %
- Vitamin B-6 16.2 %
- Vitamin C 30.6 %
- Vitamin D 0.0 %
- Vitamin E 1.1 %
- Calcium 7.3 %
- Copper 10.7 %
- Folate 14.9 %
- Iron 18.1 %
- Magnesium 11.2 %
- Manganese 18.5 %
- Niacin 16.5 %
- Pantothenic Acid 3.8 %
- Phosphorus 18.5 %
- Riboflavin 13.9 %

- Selenium 15.2 %
- Thiamin 10.1 %
- Zinc 19.0 %

*Percent Daily Values are based on a 2,000 calorie diet. Your daily values may be higher or lower depending on your calorie needs

Ingredients

- 7 tablespoons of canola or vegetable oil
- 4 pounds of beef cut into ½ inch cubes
- Salt and freshly ground pepper
- 2 tablespoons of ground cumin
- 1 ounce bottle of dark beer
- 1 large red onion (diced)
- 4 cloves of garlic
- 1 teaspoon of chopped habanero peppers
- 1 chopped Thai bird chili
- ½ of a jalapeno pepper
- ½ poblano pepper seeded and chopped
- 1 tablespoon of chili powder
- 1 tablespoon of cascabel chili powder
- 1 tablespoon of chipotle pepper puree
- 1 tablespoon of pasilla chili powder
- 1 teaspoon of New Mexican chili powder
- 5 cups of homemade chicken stock
- 1 16 ounce can of drained puréed tomatoes
- 2 tablespoons of finely chopped semi-sweet chocolate
- 2 tablespoons of maple syrup

Method of preparation

Heat 2 tablespoons of the oil in a large Dutch oven over high heat. Sprinkle the beef with salt and pepper and add one-third of the meat to the pan and sauté until browned on all sides. Repeat with the oil and meat, draining any excess liquid from the pan between the batches. Return the meat to the pan, sprinkle with the cumin and stir well. Deglaze the pan with the beer and bring to a boil. Cook until the beer is almost completely reduced. Remove the meat from the pan and set aside. In the same pan, add the remaining 1 tablespoon oil to the same pan and then add the onions and cook on medium heat until soft. Add the garlic and cook for 2 minutes. Add the habanero, Thai bird, jalapeno and poblano peppers and cook until soft, about 5 minutes. Add the chili pepper, cascabel chili powder, chipotle pepper puree, pasilla chili powder and New Mexican chili powder, and cook an additional 2 minutes. Add the chicken stock and tomatoes bring to a boil and cook until slightly thickened, 15 to 20 minutes. Puree with an immersion blender. Add the beef back to the pan reduce the heat to medium, cover and simmer until the chili is thick and the beef is tender, about 1 hour 15 minutes.

SLOW COOKER BOSTON BUTT

Nutritional value

Amount per 100 g.

- Calories 194.5
- Total Fat 9.2 g
- Saturated Fat 2.5 g
- Polyunsaturated Fat 2.5 g
- Monounsaturated Fat 3.7 g
- Cholesterol 13.8 mg
- Sodium 472.5 mg
- Potassium 828.7 mg
- Total Carbohydrate 7.7 g
- Dietary Fiber 2.6 g
- Sugars 1.2 g
- Protein 21.2 g
- Vitamin A 22.1 %
- Vitamin B-12 8.9 %
- Vitamin B-6 11.4 %
- Vitamin C 26.3 %
- Vitamin D 3.3 %
- Vitamin E 15.0 %
- Calcium 10.9 %
- Copper 14.3 %
- Folate 38.1 %
- Iron 22.4 %
- Magnesium 9.3 %
- Manganese 17.2 %
- Niacin 13.5 %
- Pantothenic Acid 39.5 %
- Phosphorus 27.0 %
- Riboflavin 37.3 %

- Selenium 53.9 %
- Thiamin 28.9 %
- Zinc 17.0 %

*Percent Daily Values are based on a 2,000 calorie diet

Ingredients

- 4-5 pound Boston butt roast
- 1 tablespoon of chili powder
- 1 tablespoon of paprika
- 1 tablespoon of garlic powder
- 1 tablespoon of sea salt
- 1 of celery salt
- 1 tablespoon of basil
- 1 teaspoon of black pepper
- ¼ cup of apple cider vinegar
- 2 cups of barbecue sauce

Method of preparation

Thinly slice the onions and place them in the bottom of a 6-quart or larger slow cooker. Rinse the Boston butt and place it on top of the onions and sprinkle with spices. Pour the whole can of pineapple over it and add the apple cider vinegar. Put the lid on the slow cooker and cook on low for 10-12 hours or until fork tender. Don't open until at least 8 hours and then check for tenderness.

SWEET AND SPICY PORK TENDERLOIN

Nutritional value

Amount per 100 g.

- Calories 143
- % Daily Value*
- Total Fat 3.5 g 5%
- Saturated fat 1.2 g 6%
- Polyunsaturated fat 0.5 g
- Monounsaturated fat 1.3 g
- Trans fat 0 g
- Cholesterol 73 mg 24%
- Sodium 57 mg 2%
- Potassium 421 mg 12%
- Total Carbohydrate 0 g 0%
- Dietary fiber 0 g 0%
- Sugar 0 g
- Protein 26 g 52%
- Vitamin A 0%
- Vitamin C 0%
- Calcium 0%
- Iron 6%
- Vitamin D 2%
- Vitamin B-6 35%
- Cobalamin 10%
- Magnesium 7%

*Per cent Daily Values are based on a 2,000 calorie diet.

Ingredients

- 2 tablespoons of chili powder
- 1 teaspoon of smoked paprika
- 1 teaspoon of salt

- ½ teaspoon of pepper
- 2 pork tenderloins
- ¼ cup of ketchup
- 2 teaspoons of apple cider vinegar
- 1 ½ teaspoon of sugar
- 1 tablespoon of vegetable oil

Method of preparation

Adjust the oven rack to the middle position and preheat the oven to 450 degrees F. Pat the pork tenderloin dry. Combine chili powder, paprika, salt and pepper. Take a tablespoon of the mixture and keep it aside, then rub the rest on the pork tenderloin on all sides. In a large non-stick pan, heat the oil over medium heat until it's very hot then add the pork and cook until all sides are brown. Transfer the pork to a baking pan pre wrapped in aluminum foil and bake. In a bowl combine the reserved mixture, ketchup and vinegar and sugar and brush over the cooked pork. Slice the pork and serve.

VIETNAMESE LAMB

Nutritional value

Amount per serving.

- Calories: 226
- % Daily Values*
- Total Fat 17.55g 27%
- Saturated Fat 7.669g 38%
- Polyunsaturated Fat 1.302g
- Monounsaturated Fat 7.186g
- Cholesterol 68mg 23%
- Sodium 281mg 12%
- Total Carbohydrate 0g 0%
- Dietary Fiber 0g 0%
- Sugars 0g
- Protein 15.86g
- Vitamin D
- Calcium 14mg 1%
- Iron 1.40mg 8%
- Potassium 184mg 5%
- Vitamin A 0IU 0%
- Vitamin C 0mg 0%

The % Daily Value (DV) tells you how much a nutrient in a serving of food contributes to a daily diet. 2,000 calories a day is used for general nutrition advice.

Ingredients

- 1 cup chopped cilantro
- 1 cup chopped mint
- ½ cup fish sauce
- ¼ cup lime juice
- ¼ cup sugar

- 1 tablespoon, chopped fresh chili (like jalapeno)
- Black pepper
- 2 pounds of lamb shoulder chops

Method of preparation

Combine, cilantro, mint, fish sauce, lime juice, sugar, chili (like jalapeño), and black pepper. Rub half of the mixture over 2 pounds of lamb shoulder chops or chunks, and marinate overnight. Heat a grill or broiler with the rack 4 to 6 inches from the flame. Wipe off the marinade; grill or broil, turning once, until medium, 4 or 5 minutes per side. Serve with the remaining sauce.

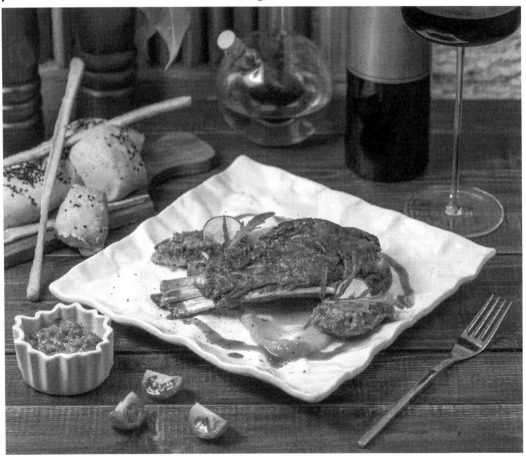

WHITE MEAT RECIPES

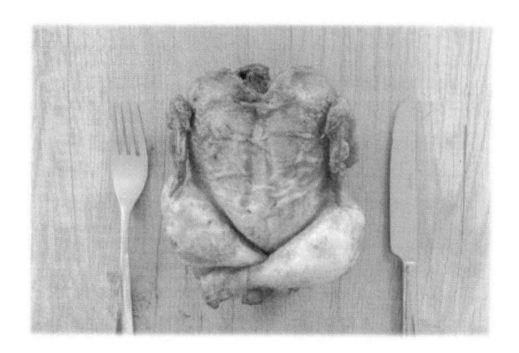

BALSAMIC CHICKEN

Ingredients

- 4 boneless skinless chicken breasts, pounded to even thickness
- Salt and pepper to taste
- ½ teaspoon Italian seasoning
- 1 cup balsamic vinegar
- ¼ cup sugar
- 1 tablespoon honey
- ½ teaspoon salt

Method of preparation

Preheat oven to 400 degrees. Season the chicken with salt, pepper, and Italian seasoning. Drizzle a pan or skillet with oil and cook chicken for 1-2 minutes on each side over medium-high heat, just to brown the very outside of the chicken. Transfer chicken to a greased baking sheet or large casserole dish. Cover with foil and bake in preheated oven for 15minutes. While chicken is cooking, make the balsamic glaze. In a small-medium sauce pan, whisk together balsamic vinegar, sugar, honey, and salt. Bring to a boil over medium-high heat, then reduce to medium-low heat and allow to simmer while the chicken is cooking. The liquid should reduce by half after 10-15 minutes. Remove from heat. Uncover chicken and brush some of the balsamic glaze on top of the chicken. Return to oven (uncovered) and bake another 5-10 minutes until chicken is completely cooked through. Drizzle remaining balsamic glaze over chicken and serve.

CARIBBEAN JERK CHICKEN

Ingredients

- 1 whole chicken
- 1 lime
- 1 large red onion
- 1 bunch green onions
- ½ teaspoon of cinnamon
- 2 teaspoons of dried thyme
- 2 teaspoons of pepper
- 2 teaspoon of salt
- 2 tablespoons of butter
- 2 teaspoons of apple cider vinegar

Method of preparation

If using a whole chicken, cut in half. Cut the lime in half and squeeze the juice over the chicken and rub it in. In a food processor (or blender) combine all remaining ingredients and process until it forms a paste. Rub the seasoning paste over the chicken halves and marinate in the refrigerator for at least a few hours or overnight. After the chicken is done marinating, preheat the oven to 375 degrees and place the chicken in a large roasting dish and place in oven. Roast for about 45 minutes to 1 hour until chicken is cooked through. Remove the chicken from the oven and serve.

CHICKEN FINGERS

Ingredients

- 3 medium chicken breasts
- 2 eggs
- 1 tsp water
- 1 cup of almond ground flax meal
- 1 teaspoon of garlic powder
- ½ teaspoon of salt
- ½ teaspoon of pepper
- 2 cups of frying oil

Method of preparation

Cut the chicken into strips or nugget size. In a medium bowl, beat eggs with 1 teaspoon of water. Add the chicken strips and toss well. In another bowl, mix together the almond ground flax meal, garlic powder, salt, and pepper. Heat the tallow or coconut oil in a large skillet over medium high heat. Once the oil is hot, remove the chicken from the egg mixture and then dredge in almond ground flax meal mixture. Place the chicken in the heated pan. Cook 3-4 minutes per side or until golden brown and cooked through. Remove from pan and keep in the oven to keep warm while additional batches are cooking. Once all are cooked through, sprinkle with additional salt and pepper and serve.

CHICKEN KATSU

Ingredients

- Chicken breasts, boneless, skinless, each about 250g
- 1 teaspoon of salt
- 1 teaspoon of ground white pepper
- A cup of almond ground flax meal to coat the chicken
- 2 eggs
- A cup of almond meal

Method of preparation

Remove the skin of the chicken breast and cut each chicken breast half into two cutlets. Season both sides of the chicken with salt and pepper and dip the chicken meat into almond ground flax meal. Remove and transfer it into beaten eggs. Turn over the meat so that both sides are wet by the eggs then, lift it and let the excess egg drip off. Dredge the chicken in almond meal but remember to remove the excess. Lightly press the surface to help the almond meal adhere to the surface. Deep fried the chicken in very hot oil and drain away the oil.

GARLIC CHICKEN

Ingredients

- ¼ cup olive
- 2 Cloves of crushed garlic
- ¼ cup of Italian seasoned almond meal
- ¼ cup of parmesan cheese
- 4 skinless boneless chicken breast halves

Method of preparation

Preheat the oven to 220 degrees C and heat olive oil and garlic in a small saucepan over low heat until warmed. Transfer garlic and oil to a shallow bowl. Add the bread crumbs and Parmesan cheese in a separate shallow bowl and dip the chicken breasts in the olive oil-garlic mixture using tongs. Transfer to bread crumb mixture and turn to evenly coat. Transfer coated chicken to a shallow baking dish. Bake in the preheated oven until no longer pink and juices run clear.

HONEY GRILLED CHICKEN THIGHS

Ingredients

- 8 boneless skinless chicken thighs
- ¼ cup of almond ground flax meal
- ¼ cup of honey or maple syrup
- 6 cloves garlic finely minced
- 1 teaspoon of salt
- ½ teaspoon of pepper

Method of preparation

Preheat the oven to 375 degrees. Place the chicken in a bowl. Sprinkle the cassava almond ground flax meal over it to coat evenly. Shake off the excess almond ground flax meal and place in a glass baking dish. In a small bowl, whisk together the honey, garlic, salt, and pepper. Pour the honey mixture evenly over the chicken. Cover lightly and bake for about 25 minutes. Remove the cover, spoon the sauce over the chicken, and bake uncovered for another 20 minutes.

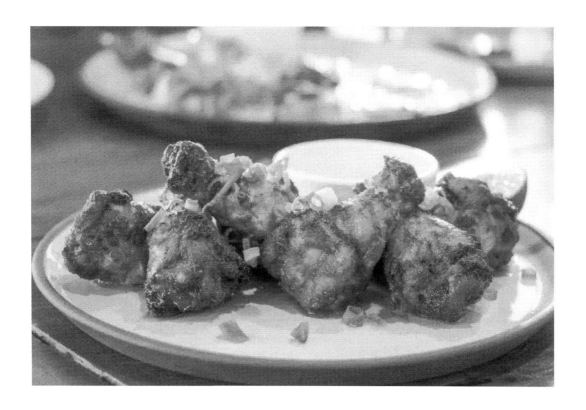

PARMESAN CHICKEN

Nutritional content

- Calories: 226
- % Daily Values*
- Total Fat 17.55g 27%
- Saturated Fat 7.669g 38%
- Polyunsaturated Fat 1.302g
- Monounsaturated Fat 7.186g
- Cholesterol 68mg 23%
- Sodium 281mg 12%
- Total Carbohydrate 0g 0%
- Dietary Fiber 0g 0%
- Sugars 0g
- Protein 15.86g
- Vitamin D
- Calcium 14mg 1%
- Iron 1.40mg 8%
- Potassium 184mg 5%
- Vitamin A 0IU 0%
- Vitamin C 0mg 0%

Ingredients

- 1 teaspoon of a clove of garlic, (minced)
- 1 stick butter, melted
- 1 cup of dried bread crumbs
- 1/3 cup of grated Parmesan cheese
- 2 tablespoon of chopped fresh parsley
- ¼ teaspoon of salt
- ¼ teaspoon of garlic salt
- A large pinch of seasoning
- 1/8 teaspoon of ground black pepper

- 2 lbs. of skinless, boneless, chicken meat, cut into 1-inch to 2-inch wide pieces

Method of preparation

Preheat oven to 450°F. Pat the chicken pieces dry with paper towels. Patting the chicken pieces dry will help the chicken pieces have crispy breading when baked. In a small bowl, stir the minced garlic into the melted butter. In another bowl mix together the almond meal, Parmesan, parsley, salt, garlic salt, seasoning, and pepper. Piece by piece, dip the chicken pieces into the garlic melted butter, and then dredge into the Parmesan breadcrumb mixture to coat. If the chicken pieces are cold, they may cause the melted butter to thicken, leaving too much butter sticking the chicken pieces. If this happens, just reheat the butter. Place coated chicken pieces on a roasting dish. Try to leave a little room between each piece. Drizzle with remaining garlic butter, until chicken is cooked through and juices run clear.

ROASTED TURKEY BREAST

Ingredients

- Turkey breast
- 5 teaspoons of lemon juice
- 1 tablespoon of olive oil
- Teaspoons of pepper
- 1 teaspoon of dried thyme
- 1 teaspoon of garlic salt
- 1 medium onion, cut into wedges
- ½ cup white wine or chicken stock

Method of preparation

Preheat oven to 325°.With fingers, carefully loosen the skin from both sides of turkey breast. Combine lemon juice and oil; brush under the skin. Combine the pepper, rosemary, thyme and garlic salt and rub it all over turkey. Place onion in a baking dish. Top with turkey breast, skin side up. Pour wine into the dish. Bake, uncovered for about 2 hours, then cover it and let stand for 15 minutes before carving.

SWEET AND SPICY CHICKEN

Ingredients

- 1 tablespoon of brown sugar
- ¼ cup of soy sauce
- 2 teaspoons of chopped ginger root
- 2 teaspoons of chopped garlic
- 2 tablespoons of hot sauce
- 2 tablespoons of honey
- 1 teaspoon of vegetable oil
- Salt and pepper to taste
- 4 skinless boneless chicken breast halves cut into ½ inch strips

Method of preparation

Mix together brown sugar, honey, soy sauce, ginger, garlic and hot sauce in a small bowl. Lightly salt and pepper the chicken strips. Heat the oil in a large pan over medium heat. Add chicken strips and brown on both sides, about 1 minute per side. Pour the sauce over the chicken. Simmer uncovered until the sauce thickens, 8 to 10 minutes and serve.

THAI CHICKEN SKEWERS

Ingredients

- ¼ cup soy sauce
- 1 teaspoon of sesame oil
- 2 tablespoon of honey
- 2 teaspoon of hot chili paste
- ½ inch fresh ginger root peeled and finely grated
- 2 cloves of garlic crushed
- 2 chicken breasts skinless and boneless

Method of preparation

Mix all marinade ingredients together. Cut chicken into cubes or chunks and thread onto skewers. Put chicken cubes in a shallow dish, pour marinade over top and turn chicken pieces to make sure all are coated or submerged. Let marinate for at least an hour in the refrigerator and grill over medium heat, turning after 7 minutes. Grill on the other side until chicken is no longer pink.

TURKEY MEATLOAF

Ingredients

- 1 lb. ground turkey (can be made in a blender)
- 1 large grated onion
- ¼ cup of almond ground flax meal
- 2 eggs
- 1 tablespoon of lemon juice
- 1 teaspoon of lemon zest
- 1 clove garlic minced
- 1 teaspoon of garlic powder
- 1 teaspoon of salt
- ½ teaspoon of pepper

Method of preparation

Preheat the oven to 350°F. In a large bowl, mix together all the ingredients for the meatloaf. Add extra almond ground flax meal if needed to make it thick enough to form into meat balls. Form into a loaf shape and place in a loaf pan or in the middle of a baking dish with a rim around the sides. Place in the preheated oven for approximately 45-60 minutes or until cooked through.

SEAFOOD RECIPES

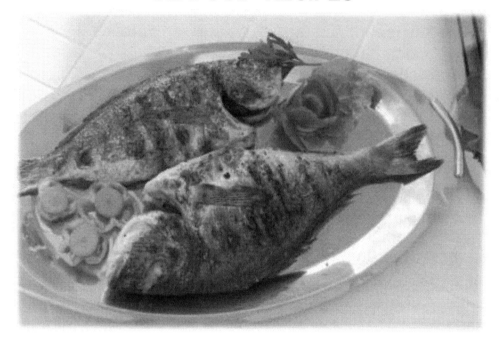

CRAB BALLS

Ingredients

- One teaspoon of salt
- One teaspoon and also one pinch of seasoning
- 1 tablespoon of finely chopped fresh parsley
- 1 tablespoon of Worcestershire sauce
- 1 cup plus 1 tablespoon of mayonnaise
- 1/3 cup of cream
- Slices crust removed and processed into crumbs bread
- 1 beaten egg
- 1 lb. picked free of any shells lump crab meat
- Frying oil
- 1 white onion
- ½ cup dill chips
- Fresh lemon juice
- Fresh ground pepper

Method of preparation

Moisten the almond meal with cream. Mix in the salt, parsley, Worcestershire, 1 tablespoon of mayonnaise, 1 egg and crab. Shape into balls about the size of a walnut. Fry in deep oil until brown. To make tartar sauce, combine 1 cup mayonnaise, onion, dill chips, lemon juice, a punch house seasoning and pepper into a food processor or a blender and blend to achieve desired chunkiness. Serve Crab Balls while hot, with tartar sauce.

CRAB CAKES

Ingredients

- Eggs that have been lightly beaten
- 8 oz. fresh lump crabmeat gently picked through and shells removed
- Two dessert spoons of lard
- One table spoon of tallow
- 1 tablespoon of mayonnaise
- 1 tablespoon of Dijon mustard
- 1 tablespoon of minced garlic
- ½ teaspoon of salt
- ½ teaspoon of dried thyme
- 1/8 teaspoon of cayenne pepper

Method of preparation

In a medium bowl, lightly whisk the egg with a fork. Mix in the crabmeat. Mix well with a fork, pressing on the crab meat with the fork and breaking up any large pieces. Mix in the mayonnaise, mustard, garlic, salt, thyme, and cayenne pepper. Then Mix in the parsley and the almond ground flax meal. Use a ¼ cup scoop to portion out six portions of the mixture. Place the crab cakes on a platter lined with wax paper. Cover loosely with plastic wrap and refrigerate for at least one hour. Heat the butter and olive oil in a large nonstick pan over medium heat, about 3 minutes. Add the crab cakes. Cook them for about 4 minutes without moving, until you can see on the edges that the bottoms are browned. Carefully, using two spatulas, flip the crab cakes. Very gently press on their tops to slightly flatten, then cook on the other side until browned, about 3-4 more minutes. Remove them to a plate lined with paper towels, then serve.

CRAB STUFFED LOBSTER TAIL

Ingredients

- 2 lobster tails, split along the center top
- 2 teaspoons of melted butter
- 15 buttery round crackers
- ½ a cup of jumbo lump crabmeat
- ¼ cup of butter
- One tablespoon of seafood seasoning
- 1 clove of garlic
- 1 teaspoon of fresh lemon juice
- 1 teaspoon of lemon zest
- 1 teaspoon of parsley
- ¼ teaspoon of salt

Method of preparation

Heat the oven to 220 degrees C and pull the edges of the split lobster shells apart and gently lift the tail meat to rest above the shells. Place the prepared lobster tails on a baking sheet. Brush each portion of tail meat with 1 teaspoon melted butter. Lightly mix the crushed crackers, crabmeat, ¼ cup of clarified butter, parsley, seafood seasoning, garlic, lemon zest, lemon juice, salt, and white pepper in a bowl until thoroughly combined. Spoon half the stuffing onto each lobster tail; press lightly to slightly shape the stuffing so it doesn't fall off. Bake the lobster tails in the preheated oven until the meat is opaque and the stuffing is golden brown on top, around 10 to 12 minutes.

FISH STICKS

Nutritional value

Amount per 100 g.

- Calories 194.5
- Total Fat 9.2 g
- Saturated Fat 2.5 g
- Polyunsaturated Fat 2.5 g
- Monounsaturated Fat 3.7 g
- Cholesterol 13.8 mg
- Sodium 472.5 mg
- Potassium 828.7 mg
- Total Carbohydrate 7.7 g
- Dietary Fiber 2.6 g
- Sugars 1.2 g
- Protein 21.2 g
- Vitamin A 22.1 %
- Vitamin B-12 8.9 %
- Vitamin B-6 11.4 %
- Vitamin C 26.3 %
- Vitamin D 3.3 %
- Vitamin E 15.0 %
- Calcium 10.9 %
- Copper 14.3 %
- Folate 38.1 %
- Iron 22.4 %
- Magnesium 9.3 %
- Manganese 17.2 %
- Niacin 13.5 %
- Pantothenic Acid 39.5 %
- Phosphorus 27.0 %
- Riboflavin 37.3 %

- Selenium 53.9 %
- Thiamin 28.9 %
- Zinc 17.0 %

*Percent Daily Values are based on a 2,000 calorie diet

Ingredients

- ½ a cup of dried almond meal
- ½ a teaspoon of salt
- ½ a teaspoon of paprika
- ½ a teaspoon of lemon pepper seasoning
- ½ a cup of all-purpose almond ground flax meal
- 1 large egg (beaten)
- ¾ pound of cod fillets cut into 1 inch strips

Method of preparation

Preheat the oven to 400 degrees. In a shallow bowl, mix almond meal and seasonings then place the almond ground flax meal and egg in another bowl. Dip the fish in the almond ground flax meal and coat both sides when done shake off the excess. Dip it in the egg then in the crumb mixture and pat it to make sure it sticks properly. Place it on a piece of aluminium foil in a baking tray coated with butter. Bake until the fish starts to flake and turn over. Do the same to the other side and serve.

LEMON BAKED COD

Nutritional value

Amount per 100 g.

- Calories 194.5
- Total Fat 9.2 g
- Saturated Fat 2.5 g
- Polyunsaturated Fat 2.5 g
- Monounsaturated Fat 3.7 g
- Cholesterol 13.8 mg
- Sodium 472.5 mg
- Potassium 828.7 mg
- Total Carbohydrate 7.7 g
- Dietary Fiber 2.6 g
- Sugars 1.2 g
- Protein 21.2 g
- Vitamin A 22.1 %
- Vitamin B-12 8.9 %
- Vitamin B-6 11.4 %
- Vitamin C 26.3 %
- Vitamin D 3.3 %
- Vitamin E 15.0 %
- Calcium 10.9 %
- Copper 14.3 %
- Folate 38.1 %
- Iron 22.4 %
- Magnesium 9.3 %
- Manganese 17.2 %
- Niacin 13.5 %
- Pantothenic Acid 39.5 %
- Phosphorus 27.0 %
- Riboflavin 37.3 %

- Selenium 53.9 %
- Thiamin 28.9 %
- Zinc 17.0 %

*Percent Daily Values are based on a 2,000 calorie diet

Ingredients

- 3 tablespoons of lemon juice
- 3 tablespoons of melted butter
- ¼ cup all-purpose almond ground flax meal
- ½ teaspoon salt
- ¼ teaspoon paprika
- 4 cod fillets (6 ounces each)
- 2 teaspoons grated lemon zest
- ¼ teaspoon of crushed garlic

Method of preparation

Preheat the oven to 400 degrees F and rub a baking sheet with melted butter. Add the rest of the butter, the lemon juice, garlic, salt and pepper in a small bowl and mix together until well combined. Spread the butter mixture evenly over each piece of salmon and bake for about 15-20 minutes or when the cod is opaque and easily flakes when turned over with a fork.

PAN FRIED SALMON

Ingredients

- 2 salmon fillets, Bones removed, skin on
- ½ teaspoon of salt
- ¼ teaspoon of black pepper
- ½ teaspoon of garlic powder
- ½ teaspoon dried rosemary
- 2 tablespoons of unsalted butter

Method of preparation

Dry the salmon fillets with paper towels. Sprinkle them with the salt, pepper, and garlic powder. Heat the butter in a large nonstick pan over medium-high heat, about 2 minutes. Add the salmon fillets, skin side down. Cook until skin is browned and crisp, about 3 minutes. Use a spatula to carefully turn the fillets. Cook until browned on the second side and cooked through, after 2-3 more minutes. Transfer the salmon to plates and pour the butter from the pan on top. Serve immediately.

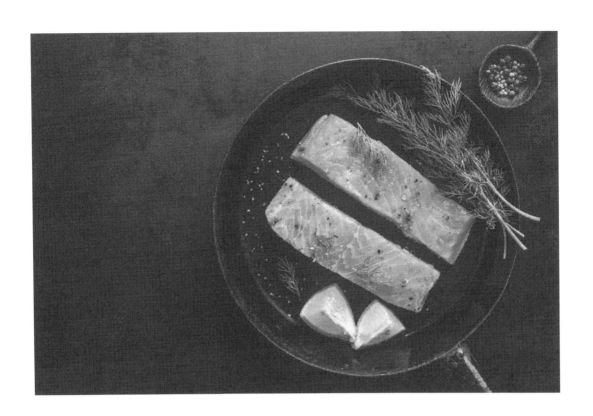

PARMESAN BAKED SHRIMP

Ingredients

- 4 tablespoons butter
- Cup grated Parmesan
- ½ teaspoon black pepper
- 1 teaspoon garlic powder
- 24 oz. jumbo shrimp peeled and deveined, patted dry
- ½ teaspoon paprika
- Avocado oil cooking spray

Method of preparation

Preheat oven to 233 degrees C. Line a rimmed baking sheet with parchment paper. Place the butter in a shallow microwave safe bowl. Melt in the microwave. In another medium bowl, whisk together the Parmesan, black pepper and garlic powder. Divide the mixture into two separate shallow bowls – this will ensure the Parmesan stays as dry as possible, making it easier to coat the shrimp. Dip each shrimp in the melted butter to coat, then roll in the Parmesan mixture. Arrange the coated shrimp in a single layer on the prepared baking sheet. Sprinkle them with paprika and spray with avocado oil. Bake the Parmesan shrimp until cooked through, about 10 minutes and serve immediately.

SEAFOOD CREOLE

Ingredients

- ¾ teaspoon of dried oregano
- ½ teaspoon of salt
- ½ teaspoon of ground white pepper
- ½ teaspoon of ground black pepper
- ½ teaspoon of cayenne pepper
- ½ teaspoon of dried thyme leaves
- ½ teaspoon of dried sweet basil
- ¼ a cup of butter
- ½ a cup of peeled chopped onion
- ¾ cup of chopped onion
- ¾ cup of chopped celery
- ¾ cup of chopped green bell peppers
- ½ teaspoon of minced garlic
- 1 ¼ cup of chicken stock
- 1 cup of canned tomato sauce
- 1 teaspoon of white sugar
- ½ teaspoon of hot pepper sauce
- Bay leaves
- 1 pound of peeled and deveined shrimp
- 1 pound of scallops
- 1 pound of haddock fillets

Method of preparation

Mix together oregano, salt, white pepper, black pepper, cayenne pepper, thyme, and basil in a small bowl; set aside. Melt butter in a large oven over medium heat; stir in tomato, onion, celery, green bell pepper, and garlic. Cook and stir until the onion is translucent, about 5 minutes. Stir in chicken stock, tomato sauce, sugar, hot pepper sauce, and bay leaves. Reduce heat to low and bring sauce to a simmer. Stir in seasoning mix and simmer until the flavors have blended, about 20 minutes. Gently stir in shrimp, scallops, and haddock; bring sauce back to a simmer and cook until the shellfish and fish are opaque, about 20 more minutes. Remove bay leaves to serve.

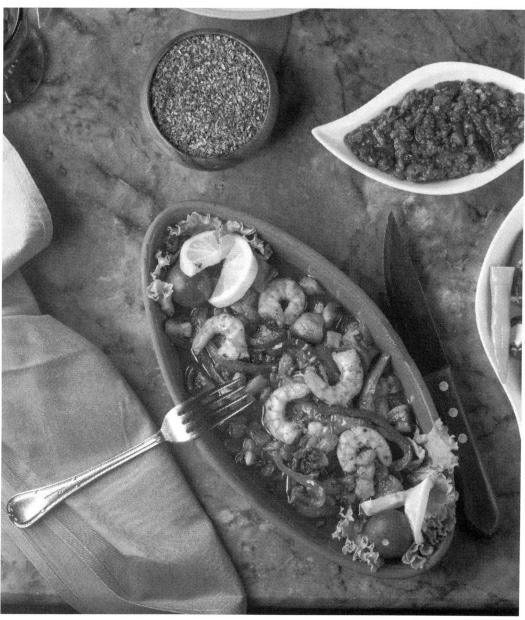

SEAFOOD SAUTEE

Ingredients

- 2 lb. frozen mixed seafood (of your choice, includes but not limited to: shrimps, lobsters, calamari, scallions etc.)
- 4 tablespoons unsalted butter, melted
- One teaspoon salt
- 1 tablespoon minced garlic
- 1 teaspoon paprika
- ½ teaspoon red pepper flakes

Method of preparation

Place the frozen seafood in a large bowl. Fill the bowl with cool water. Allow to defrost for about 5 minutes, stirring gently to separate pieces (replacing the water once during the defrosting process). Place the defrosted seafood on a clean kitchen towel or on paper towels to dry. Melt the butter in a very large skillet over medium-high heat. When foaming subsides, add the seafood, salt, minced garlic, paprika, and red pepper flakes. Stir-fry just until opaque, about 5 minutes. Transfer the sautéed seafood to a serving platter, spooning the pan juices on top and serve.

SEARED SCALLOPS

Ingredients

- 1lb sea scallop (side muscles removed)
- Fine sea salt
- Tablespoon of black pepper, freshly ground
- 1 tablespoon of extra virgin olive oil
- Tablespoons of unsalted butter cut into small pieces
- 1 of clove garlic, grated
- 1 tablespoon dry white wine

Method of preparation

Pat the scallops dry with a paper towel. Season them with salt and pepper. In a large pot set over medium-high heat, add the oil. When the oil is hot, add the scallops and cook until golden brown on one side, 2-3 minutes. Gently turn the scallops, and add the butter and garlic to the pan. Continue to cook, spooning the butter over the scallops until they are cooked through, about 3 minutes more. Add the white wine, cook another 10 seconds and serve.

SEASONED TILAPIA FILLETS

Ingredients

- 2 tilapia fillets (6 ounces each)
- 1 tablespoon of melted butter
- 1 teaspoon of steak seasoning
- ½ teaspoon of dried parsley flakes
- ¼ teaspoon of paprika
- ¼ teaspoon of dried thyme
- 1/8 teaspoon of onion powder
- 1/8 teaspoon of salt
- 1/8 teaspoon of pepper
- A dash of garlic powder

Method of preparation

Preheat oven to 425 degrees F and place the tilapia in a greased baking pan then, drizzle it with butter. In a small bowl, mix the remaining ingredients and sprinkle over the fillets. Bake it covered for 10 minutes. Uncover it then, bake until the fish just begins to flake easily.

STEAMED LOBSTER

Ingredients

- Tablespoon sea salt
- 4 lobster tails
- 125g butter, melted

Method of preparation

Fill a large pot with about 1 inch of water and bring to the boil. Add the salt and place a steamer insert inside the pot so that it is just above the water level. Place the lobster tails inside the steamer and cover the pot. Steam them for at most 8 minutes without taking off the lid. Serve with melted butter.

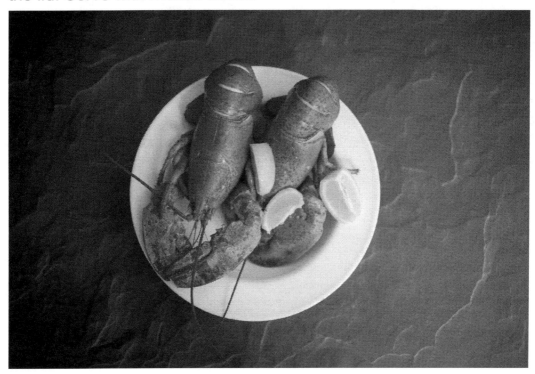

SALMON WITH BROWN SUGAR AND MUSTARD

Ingredients

- Tablespoon of extra-virgin olive oil
- 1 large shallot
- ¼ cup of red-wine vinegar
- ¼ cup of Dijon mustard
- ¼ cup of dark brown sugar
- ½ a tablespoon of salt
- ½ tablespoon of ground pepper
- 1 side salmon about 3 pounds (cut into 8 fillets)
- 1 lemon

Method of preparation

Heat your oven to 400 degrees and add salt and pepper to the salmon fillets. Place the salmon fillets skin-side down on a lightly oiled, foil-lined baking sheet. Make a mixture of Dijon mustard and brown sugar to the degree of spicy-sweetness that pleases you Slather the tops of the fillets with the mustard and brown sugar glaze and slide them into the top half of your oven. Roast for about 12 minutes and serve.

TUNA PATTIES

Ingredients

- 2 tablespoons of butter
- 3 tablespoons of all-purpose almond ground flax meal
- 1 cup of evaporated milk
- 5 ounces of light tuna in water
- ½ cup dry bread crumbs
- 1 green onion, finely chopped
- 2 tablespoons lemon juice
- ½ teaspoon salt
- ¼ teaspoon pepper
- Oil for frying

Method of preparation

In a small saucepan, melt butter over medium heat. Stir in almond ground flax meal until smooth; gradually whisk in milk. Bring to a boil, stirring constantly. Cook and stir until thickened, then remove from heat. Transfer to a small bowl and let it cool down. Stir in tuna, 1/3 cup bread crumbs, lemon juice, salt and pepper. Refrigerate, covered, at least 30 minutes. Place remaining ½ cup bread crumbs in a shallow bowl. Drop 1/3 cup tuna mixture into crumbs. Gently coat and shape into a ½ inch thick patty. In a large pan, heat oil over medium heat. Add tuna patties in batches and cook until golden brown, 2-3 minutes on each side. Place them on paper towels to drain and serve.

ORGAN MEAT RECIPES

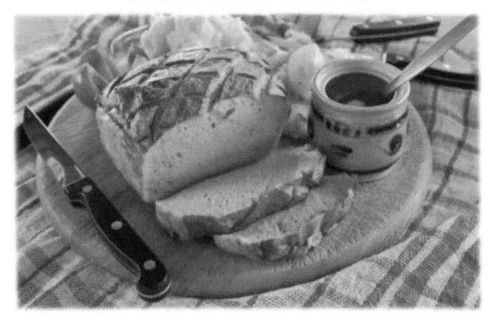

LIVER WITH LEMON THYME

Ingredients

- Lb. calves liver
- Tablespoon olive oil
- 10 sprigs fresh lemon thyme, chopped
- Salt and pepper to taste

Method of preparation

First, rinse the liver and pat dry. Then, with a sharp knife, remove any exposed veins, ducts or connective tissue. Next, use your fingers to remove the thin outer membrane, being careful not to tear the liver itself. From there, slice the liver into about ¼ inch thick slices. Rinse again and pat dry. Next, heat olive oil in a large pot over medium heat. Add the fresh thyme to the pan, and then lay the liver on top. Cook over medium heat for about 4 minutes, then flip and cook on other side the liver should be eaten slightly pink, so take care not to overcook as it can make the liver tough. Season it with salt and pepper as desired and serve.

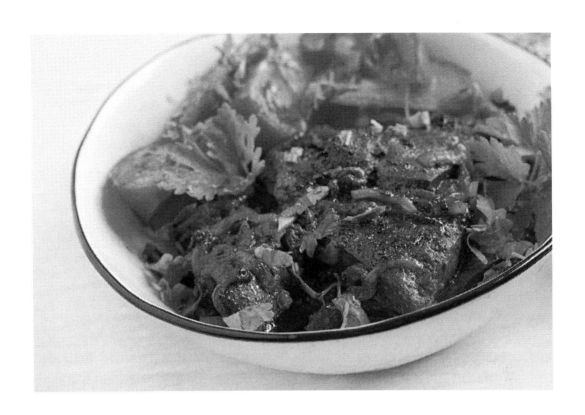

PERFECT PATE

Ingredients

- 6 tablespoons of butter
- ½ cup onion finely minced
- 1 clove garlic finely minced
- ½ lb. of chicken liver
- ½ teaspoon of salt
- ½ teaspoon of pepper
- ½ teaspoon of dried thyme
- 3 tablespoon of apple cider vinegar
- 2 tablespoons of cream

Method of preparation

In a medium size pan, melt 3 tablespoons of the butter. Add the finely minced onion and garlic and cook on medium until translucent- 3-4 minutes. Meanwhile, trim the connective tissue off of the livers. Add the livers to the pan and sprinkle with salt, pepper, and thyme. Brown livers for 6-10 minutes until cooked on the outside and barely pink on the inside. Add the apple cider vinegar and cook until it thickens, 2-3 minutes. Remove the pan from the heat and let it cool for about 5 minutes. Put the livers in a blender and puree until smooth. While blending/pureeing, add the remaining butter and cream if using. Add more salt and pepper to taste, if desired. Once mixture is completely smooth, remove it from blender and put in a glass container and cover tightly. Put in the refrigerator overnight to harden and let the flavors meld.

SAUTEED KIDNEYS IN RED WINE SAUCE

Ingredients

- Lb. lamb kidneys
- ¼ cup wine vinegar
- Tablespoons of butter
- Tablespoons of olive oil
- ½ medium onion, finely diced
- 1 cup of mushrooms, cleaned and sliced
- ¼ cup red wine
- Salt and pepper to taste

Method of preparation

To prepare kidneys for cooking, first rinse and pat dry. With a sharp knife, remove the outside membrane, cut in half, and remove any white fat and tubes from center. Place in the bottom of a medium bowl, cover with cold water and ¼ cup of wine vinegar. Let it soak for half an hour. Remove from solution, rinse and pat dry. In a pan, melt the butter and oil and lightly brown the kidneys. Remove and set aside. Next, add the onion and mushrooms to the pan and cook, stirring frequently, until onion becomes near translucent. Add the wine and cook for another minute or so. Return kidneys to pan heat through and serve immediately.

SPICY MARINATED CHICKEN LIVER AND GIZZARD

Nutritional value

Amount per serving.

- Calories 194.5
- Total Fat 9.2 g
- Saturated Fat 2.5 g
- Polyunsaturated Fat 2.5 g
- Monounsaturated Fat 3.7 g
- Cholesterol 13.8 mg
- Sodium 472.5 mg
- Potassium 828.7 mg
- Total Carbohydrate 7.7 g
- Dietary Fiber 2.6 g
- Sugars 1.2 g
- Protein 21.2 g
- Vitamin A 22.1 %
- Vitamin B-12 8.9 %
- Vitamin B-6 11.4 %
- Vitamin C 26.3 %
- Vitamin D 3.3 %
- Vitamin E 15.0 %
- Calcium 10.9 %
- Copper 14.3 %
- Folate 38.1 %
- Iron 22.4 %
- Magnesium 9.3 %
- Manganese 17.2 %
- Niacin 13.5 %
- Pantothenic Acid 39.5 %
- Phosphorus 27.0 %
- Riboflavin 37.3 %

- Selenium 53.9 %
- Thiamin 28.9 %
- Zinc 17.0 %

*Percent Daily Values are based on a 2,000 calorie diet

Ingredients

- 2 chicken livers, (cut)
- 2 chicken gizzard, (cut)
- 2 green chilies, sliced diagonally
- ¼ teaspoon coriander powder
- Sugar and salt (to your taste)
- Ground spices (cumin, jalapeño, curry, rosemary, thyme etc.)
- 2 cloves of garlic
- 3 small red onions
- 7 cayenne peppers

Method of preparation

Stir-fry all spices until fragrant Add the chicken liver and gizzard, cook until cooked and add a little water to aid the cooking process. Then add in the green chilies and coriander powder. Cook until the chili is wilted. Shortly before finishing, put in the sugar and salt, stir and simmer briefly then serve.

VEAL KIDNEYS FLAMBE

Ingredients

- 6 veal kidneys, trimmed and cut into thin slices
- 2 cups of milk for soaking
- ½ cup of shallots, peeled and finely chopped
- 2 cups of mushrooms
- 1 tablespoon of vinegar
- 1 cup of melted salted butter
- 1 tablespoon of cracked pepper
- ½ cup brandy, (warmed)
- 1 cup cream
- Salt to taste

Method of preparation

Soak trimmed kidneys in milk at room temperature for about an hour. Remove and pat dry. In a frying pan, sauté mushrooms and shallots in butter. Remove to a heated platter and keep warm. Add more butter to the pan and when it foams, sauté the kidney slices in batches. Add the vinegar to the pan and then the brandy. Light the brandy and let it flambé. When the flame disappears, add the cream and pepper. Bring to the boil and let the sauce reduce a bit and season to taste with salt. Serve the kidney slices on heated plates garnished with shallot-mushroom mixture and a spoonful of the sauce.

Made in the USA
Las Vegas, NV
18 July 2024

92530592R00085